WORKBOOK TO ACCOMPANY

NURSING ASSISTING

Essentials for Long-Term Care

Second Edition

WORKBOOK TO ACCOMPANY

NURSING ASSISTING

Essentials for Long-Term Care

Second Edition

Barbara Acello, MS, RN
Independent Nurse Consultant and Educator

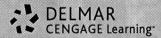

DELMAR
CENGAGE Learning

Australia • Brazil • Japan • Korea • Mexico • Singapore • Spain • United Kingdom • United States

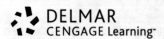

**Workbook to Accompany, Nursing Assisting:
Essentials for Long-Term Care,
Second Edition**
Barbara Acello

Vice President, Health Care Business Unit:
    William Brottmiller

Editorial Director: Cathy L. Esperti

Acquisitions Editor: Marah E. Bellegarde

Developmental Editor: Sherry Conners

Marketing Director: Jennifer McAvey

Marketing Channel Manager: Tamara Caruso

Marketing Coordinator: Kip Summerlin

Project Editor: Daniel Branagh

Production Coordinator: Jessica McNavich

Art and Design Specialists: Connie
    Lundberg-Watkins Alexandros Vasilako

For product information and technology assistance, contact us at
Cengage Learning Customer & Sales Support, 1-800-354-9706

For permission to use material from this text or product,
submit all requests online at **www.cengage.com/permissions**
Further permissions questions can be emailed to
permissionrequest@cengage.com

ISBN-13: 978-1-4018-6494-1

ISBN-10: 1-4018-6494-5

Delmar
Executive Woods
5 Maxwell Drive
Clifton Park, NY 12065
USA

Cengage Learning is a leading provider of customized learning solutions with office locations around the globe, including Singapore, the United Kingdom, Australia, Mexico, Brazil, and Japan. Locate your local office at **international.cengage.com/region**

Cengage Learning products are represented in Canada by Nelson Education, Ltd.

For your lifelong learning solutions, visit **www.cengage.com/delmar**

Visit our corporate website at **www.cengage.com**

Notice to the Reader
Publisher does not warrant or guarantee any of the products described herein or perform any independent analysis in connection with any of the product information contained herein. Publisher does not assume, and expressly disclaims, any obligation to obtain and include information other than that provided to it by the manufacturer. The reader is expressly warned to consider and adopt all safety precautions that might be indicated by the activities described herein and to avoid all potential hazards. By following the instructions contained herein, the reader willingly assumes all risks in connection with such instructions. The publisher makes no representations or warranties of any kind, including but not limited to, the warranties of fitness for particular purpose or merchantability, nor are any such representations implied with respect to the material set forth herein, and the publisher takes no responsibility with respect to such material. The publisher shall not be liable for any special, consequential, or exemplary damages resulting, in whole or part, from the readers' use of, or reliance upon, this material.

Printed in the United States of America
    2 3 4 5 6   13 12 11 10 09

ED320

Contents

Preface

The content of your workbook follows a basic organizational pattern. Each lesson begins with the key points from the corresponding textbook chapter. Review these first before proceeding to the activities. Each chapter has activities covering the vocabulary terms and other important content. These exercises will help you review, recall, reinforce, and apply the material from each chapter. Complete the workbook while the information is fresh in your mind. Students who complete activities such as these perform better, have more confidence in their abilities, and are more secure in the basic concepts than those who do not.

The development of critical thinking skills should be a lifelong quest for health care personnel. Critical thinking involves having knowledge and skills to process and generate information and beliefs, and the practice of using this information to guide your behavior and benefit the residents. Critical thinking involves actively and skillfully conceptualizing, applying, analyzing, synthesizing, and/or evaluating information gathered from, or generated by, observation, experience, reflection, reasoning, or communication, as a guide to belief and action (Scriven & Paul, 2003).

You will also receive many personal and professional benefits from critical thinking. The information in your textbook provides the basic foundation information you will need to think critically in your nursing assistant role. The exercises and activities in this workbook help you learn to apply this information and become a critical thinker! You can make the best use of this information by:

- Reading and studying the related chapter in the text and doing the exercise at the end of that chapter.

- Observing and listening carefully to your instructor's explanations and demonstrations.

- Reviewing the chapter objectives at the beginning of each chapter when you begin the lesson. Review them a second time after completing all the activities to ensure that you have met them. Objectives map out the important points that you will learn in each chapter. Objectives are tools used to measure learning. They describe student behavior, performance, knowledge, and information gained as a result of the learning experience. Objectives are used to make judgments about learning. There are many types of objectives. Many of the objectives for the nursing assistant are *behavioral objectives*. These describe behavior students must demonstrate or perform to show that learning took place. Because learning cannot be seen directly, the instructor must make inferences from evidence he or she can see and measure. Likewise, you should use the objectives to measure your own learning.

- Carefully studying the vocabulary words in each chapter so you understand their meaning and learn how to spell them. You will need to know these vocabulary words to understand chapter content and work in the health care field. These words are highlighted in your text and defined at their first use. The meanings are summarized in a glossary at the end of the book, which lists the terms and their meanings in alphabetical order for quick reference.

- Using the key points to quickly review and reinforce chapter content. The key points are a summary of important information presented in each chapter.

■ Completing the activities in this workbook. Circle the numbers of any that you do **not understand**. Discuss these with your instructor the next day.

It is the author's sincere desire that this workbook will offer you support and assistance **in learning** and applying critical thinking. Becoming a nursing assistant is a very special goal. Realize that to **attain this** goal, you must take many small steps. Each step you master takes you closer to your ultimate goal.

Barbara Acello

Adapted from Scriven, M. and Paul, S. *Defining critical thinking; a draft statement.* Retrieved from http://www.criticalthinking.org/University/univclass/Defining.html. Accessed 12 December 2003.

Tips on Studying Effectively

THE LEARNING PROCESS

Students may feel anxious about the learning process. Learning about health care is usually very different from other types of learning. Learning does not have to be a chore. In fact, it can be very pleasurable and rewarding if you have an open mind, a desire to succeed, and a willingness to follow some simple steps. You have already won half the battle by enrolling in the nursing assistant program. This shows that you are willing and ready to accomplish a commendable, real-life goal: becoming a nursing assistant.

Steps to Learning

There are three main steps to learning:

- Active listening
- Effective studying
- Careful practice and application of the information

Students remember

- 10% of what they read
- 20% of what they hear
- 30% of what they see
- 50% of what they see and hear
- 70% of what they say
- 90% of what they see and do concurrently when performing a skill or doing homework, papers, or assignments

Active Listening

Listening actively is not easy, natural, or passive. It is, however, a skill that can be learned and mastered. In fact, mastering active listening will help you in many ways in both your career and your personal life. Good listeners are not born that way. They are made. In fact, they work hard to master this skill. Eventually, it becomes a part of them. The average listening efficacy in our culture is about 20% to 25%. This means that although you may hear (a passive action) all that is being said, you actually listen to and process about a fourth of the material. Effective listening requires a conscious effort on the part of the listener. The most neglected communication skill is listening.

An important part of your work involves listening to residents and coworkers. To master this skill, begin to listen actively to your instructor. Hearing but not processing the information puts you and the residents in jeopardy. Active listening requires listening with personal involvement. The three actions involved are

- hearing what is said (a passive action)
- processing the information (active action)
- applying and using the information (active action)

Hearing What Is Said.   People speak an average of 125 words a minute. You must pay close attention to hear what a speaker has said. This is not difficult if you do not let other thoughts and sounds interfere with your thinking. If you sit up straight and lean forward in the classroom, or stand erect in the clinical area, your whole body is more receptive. Position yourself where you can adequately see, hear, and focus on what is being said. Make eye contact if possible, and remain alert.

Many distractions can break your concentration unless you take action to prevent them from doing so. For example, distractions may be

- interruptions, such as noise or movement in the classroom or resident's unit.
- daydreaming or thinking about personal activities, plans, or problems.
- fatigue caused by inadequate sleep and rest.
- hunger, thirst, or other discomfort.
- lack of interest because you cannot see the immediate importance of or need for the information.

To become an active listener, you must consciously work on eliminating these distractions and staying focused on the information being presented.

Processing the Information.   Remember that hearing the words is not enough. You must process them actively by making sense of them in your brain. This is called *processing*. Putting meaning to them takes effort. Here are some things you can do to help the process:

- Interact with the speaker by making eye contact, smiling, and nodding.
- Ask meaningful questions. Contribute your own comments during class discussions.
- Take notes and review them.

These actions enable your memory to establish relationships to previously learned knowledge and to make new connections.

Notetaking is another skill that can be learned and mastered. Taking notes is a good way to imprint what you are processing. You are not only hearing the sounds of the words, but also seeing them on paper. Here are some tips for making this task easier:

- Come prepared with pencil and paper.
- Do not try to write down every word.
- Write down only the important points or key words.
- Listen carefully to the beginning of the sentence, which usually reveals the primary purpose.
- Pay close attention to the final statement, which is often a summary.

Outlines include the important points summarized in a meaningful way. Be sure to leave room so you can add material. There are different ways of outlining. One way is to use letters and numbers to designate important points (Figure 1). Another is to draw a pattern of lines to show relationships (Figure 2). Use either way or one of your own design, but be consistent. Practice helps you master the skill of outlining.

When making notes, mark material that is important or unclear. For example, place a star (*) by important material, and circle the number of things that need clarification. Get unclear material clarified when the instructor asks for questions. When studying, pay close attention to the information you have marked. If the instructor stresses a point, underline it. This will call special attention to the material when you are studying. After class, reorganize your notes and add information from the text, if necessary. Make additional notes when doing your class lessons and reading assignments, if this helps you in studying.

```
I. Textbook organization
   A. Title
      1. Gives topic
      2. Sets frame of reference
   B. Objectives
      1. Direct learning
      2. Read before and after studying
   C. Vocabulary
      1. Explained in lesson
      2. Defined in glossary
   D. Body of text
      1. Simple language
      2. Explains important concepts
      3. Explains procedures
   E. End Unit materials
      1. Test learning
      2. Provide practice
```

FIGURE 1 In this form of outlining, letters and numbers are used to show the important points.

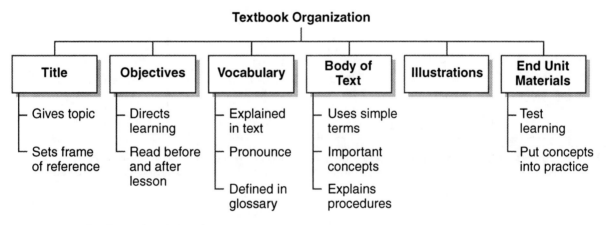

FIGURE 2 In this form of outlining, lines connect important points.

The Study Plan and Life Balance

Plan a schedule for study (Figure 3). Sit down and write a weekly schedule, hour by hour, so you know exactly how your time is being spent. Then plan and schedule specific study times—but be realistic. Study must be balanced with your other activities. Experts say that for greatest fulfillment, your life must be balanced. Look at Figure 4A. Using a 1 to 10 scale, honestly mark your satisfaction with each piece of the circle on Figure 4C, so it looks somewhat similar to Figure 4B. This will give you a good idea of areas in which your life needs more balance or fulfillment.

Learn to budget your time so that you have regular study and preparation time. You may need to block in extra time for tests or special projects. Make sure you block in time for fun and relaxation as well. Look back over your week to see how well you have adhered to your schedule. If you had difficulty, readjust the schedule to better meet your needs. If you have been successful, pat yourself on the back. You have done a great job!

Steps to Planning
I.   Block in the hours that are routine first (e.g., class hours, times to get children to school, clinical days)
II.   Don't forget to allow travel time if needed
III. Plan responsibilities that must be met daily/weekly (e.g., food shopping, banking, church attendance, and other hour limitations)
IV.   Plan daily study time
V.   Plan regular recreation time
VI.   Reevaluate plan after the first week and make necessary adjustments

Date	Hour	7 Day Planning Calendar						
		Mon	Tues	Wed	Thur	Fri	Sat	Sun
	6–7 am							
	7–8							
	8–9							
	9–10							
	10–11							
	11–12							
	12–1							
	1–2							
	2–3							
	3–4							
	4–5							
	5–6							
	6–7							
	7–8							
	8–9							
	9–10							
	10–11							
	11–12							

FIGURE 3 Write a weekly schedule, hour by hour. Analyze it to see how you are using your time. Block out a realistic time period for study. You deserve this time to invest in yourself, your future, and your career

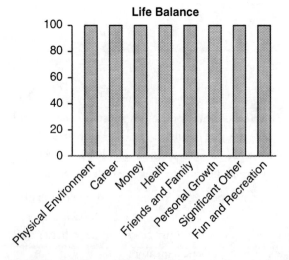

FIGURE 4A If your life is well balanced, each section takes an equal amount of time and energy.

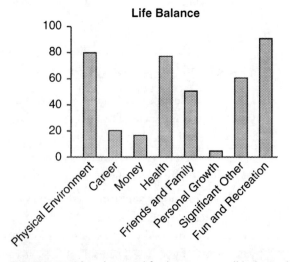

FIGURE 4B This shows a life that is not well balanced. If your life is out of balance, you have a bumpy road.

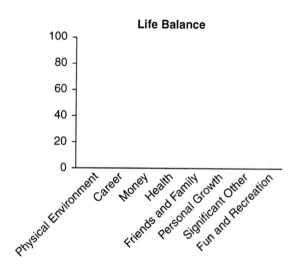

FIGURE 4C Use this chart to identify areas of your life that need balance. Draw a line showing the time and energy devoted to each area of your life.

Try to make your study area special. It does not have to be fancy. You should have enough light to see well, and a desk or table to work on. Have a supply of paper and pencils. Sharpen the pencils at the end of each study period and have paper ready for the next session. This may sound odd, but time is often wasted at the beginning of study sessions finding what you need. If these things are ready when you sit down, you can begin without distractions. Keep a medical dictionary and other study aids in your study area. When you get home, put your text and workbook there. Your work area is specifically for study. When you sit down, you will be physically and psychologically prepared to study.

Class Study. Now that you have your study area and schedule organized, think about how you can get the most from your class experience.

■ Before class, get a good night's sleep and eat a balanced meal.

■ Come prepared. Read the objectives and lesson before class. This familiarizes you with the focus of the lesson and vocabulary.

■ Come to class prepared, willing, and anxious to learn. Your success is affected by your attitude toward learning.

■ Listen actively to what the instructor is saying. If your mind starts to wander, refocus immediately.

■ Take notes on special points. Use these to study at home.

■ Participate in class activities and discussions. These subjects have been selected because they relate to the lesson. You can learn much by listening to others' comments and by contributing comments of your own.

■ Pay attention to teaching aids such as videos, transparencies, and posters. These provide a visual approach to the subject. You may wish to make notes of important points.

■ Ask intelligent and pertinent questions. Make sure your questions are simple and focused on the topic. Jot down the answers for later study.

■ Use models and charts, when available. Study them and see how they apply to the lesson.

■ Carefully observe your instructor's demonstrations. Each state has acceptable methods of performing each procedure. Your instructor will inform you if the sequence in your state differs from the procedure listed in your text. Note state-specific changes in your book or skills checklists.

- Carefully practice skills and perform return demonstrations. Remember, these are real skills you will be using on residents in the clinical area.

After Class.   After class is over, take a break. This will refresh you so you will be ready to settle down and study. You can gain the most from the experience by

- studying in your prepared study area. Everything will be ready and waiting for you if you followed the first part of the plan.

- reading over the lesson, beginning with the behavioral objectives.

- using a highlighter, pen, or pencil to mark important material.

- answering the questions at the end of the chapter. Check any that you found difficult or answered incorrectly by reviewing that section of the text.

- completing the related workbook lesson.

- reviewing the behavioral objectives at the beginning of the chapter. Ask yourself if you have met them. If not, go back and review.

- preparing the next day's lesson or assignment.

- using the medical dictionary to look up words that are not in the glossary. The dictionary will help you learn how to pronounce words you are unsure of.

Study Groups.   Group learning involves using shared and learned information, values, resources, and ways of doing things. Groups become successful by combining all these factors. Each group and each individual is only as effective as the members are willing to embrace and respect differences within the group. Groups are most effective when members respect and encourage one another and have common goals and a commitment to learning the material. Studying with someone else who is trying to learn the material is very helpful and supportive, but there are some pitfalls you must avoid

- Limit the number of people studying to no more than three; one other person is best.

- Stay focused on the subject. Do not talk about classmates or the day's social events.

- Come prepared for the study session. Have your work completed. Use the study session to reinforce your learning and develop a deeper understanding of the material.

- Ask each other questions about the materials.

- Practice and use your active listening skills in your study group.

- Make a list of questions to ask the instructor.

- Limit the study session to a specific length of time.

Group members should:

- develop and share common goals.

- contribute to the group by sharing their understanding of the material, information, problems, questions, and solutions.

- respond to, and try to understand, others' questions, insights, and solutions.

- share their strengths and help others understand the source of those strengths.

Practice your procedure skills in your study group and have others critique you. Your instructor will evaluate your skills throughout your class. Others will watch you performing these skills in the clinical area. Practicing the skills in your study group will help you become comfortable with the procedures and confident in your ability to do them correctly. It will also help you overcome the nervousness and self-consciousness you feel when someone is watching you and evaluating your performance.

Each member empowers the others to speak and contribute. Members are accountable to one another. As a group member, you must learn to depend on others, but they also must be able to depend on you. The mutual respect, giving, taking, and sharing are the things that make a successful study group.

General Tips.   The following are some general tips to help you study and master the material:

- Review the objectives when you begin to study. They are like a roadmap that will take you to your goal. Feel certain that each lesson you master is important in preparing your knowledge and skills. The workbook, textbook, and instructor materials have been carefully coordinated to meet the objectives. Read the objectives again when you have finished studying to verify that each has been met.

- Take responsibility for studying and take credit for your success. The instructor is your guide and the written materials are your tools. Using these things wisely is your responsibility. If you do so, you deserve credit for being successful!

- Take an honest look at yourself and your study habits. Take positive steps to avoid habits that could limit your success. For example, do you let your family responsibilities or social opportunities interfere with study times? If so, sit down with them and plan a study schedule that they will support. Adhere to this schedule. Find a quiet, distraction-free place to study. If the phone rings, take it off the hook or unplug it. Let everyone know this is your study time. Studying is an investment in your future. Finding time to do it may be a sacrifice for everyone. Remember, it is a short-term sacrifice with long-term dividends. You are worth the investment!

- Follow your study plan and you will succeed!

An excellent guide with many tips on learning to study, classroom participation, preparing for and taking tests, and learning in study groups is available online at http://www.studygs.net.

Avoiding Procrastination.   *Procrastination* is putting off or delaying something needlessly or unnecessarily. It is a bad habit for some people. To remedy procrastination, start with one project or lesson. If you are not sure how to reach your goal, discuss it with your instructor and ask for help or advice.
Examine your attitude:

- Do you think this is just too difficult?

- Do you feel inadequate to meet the challenges of this class?

- Do you believe you cannot function without a lot of approval?

- Are you frustrated with the limitations of others?

- Do you expect nothing less of yourself and others than perfection?

- Are you convinced that disaster hinges on your actions?

These are all self-defeating, paralyzing, procrastination-producing attitudes and beliefs. Recognize them for what they are. Do not believe them and do not indulge in them! Replace them with positive, self-enhancing beliefs and attitudes. When negative thoughts sneak in, force them out with positive thinking, such as:

- I can do this. I am doing this.

- I am doing well with this. I have mastered _____.

- I can make the time for this and I can accomplish my goal.

The objective is to avoid wallowing in self-defeating thoughts and behavior by replacing them with positive thoughts and behavior. Over time, the positives will become a part of you, permanently replacing the negatives. Answer these questions:

- What do you want to do?

- What is the final objective of this project or lesson?

- What are the major steps to getting it done? (Answer this question in general. Do not get too detailed.)
- What have you done so far? (Remind yourself that you are part of the way there, even if it is just through thinking about it. Remember, the longest journey begins with the very first step!)
- Why do you want to do this?
- What is your greatest motivation for doing this? (Be honest. If your motivation is negative, reword it until it is written positively.)
- What positive results will you gain from achieving this goal? (Identifying these will help you discover hidden benefits that you may be avoiding. Dare to dream! List everything that stands in your way.)
- What is in your power to change?
- What outside resources do you need, if any? (Resources can include physical items, such as tools, money, time, people, and attitude.)
- What will happen if you do not progress?

Next, develop a plan.

- List major, realistic steps. Start small. A project is much easier when you begin with little steps. Add detail and complexity as you achieve and grow. Concentrate on small parts. Avoid thinking of it as an all-or-nothing affair.
- How much time each will step take? Develop a realistic schedule that will help you chart your progress.
- Identify specific study times that you will devote to yourself. This helps you develop a new habit of working, build a good work environment, and fend off distractions. (It is much easier to enjoy your project when distractions are set aside.)
- List how you will reward yourself at each milestone. Identify things that you will deny yourself until you reach the milestone.
- Schedule time for review. Ask a spouse, relative, or friend to help you stay motivated and monitor your progress.

Admit to

- false starts and mistakes as learning experiences. These can be as important as successes. Admitting to them gives meaning to experience.
- temptations. Do not deny they exist.
- emotions, including frustration when things do not go well

Next,

- admit that you have had a problem, but also that you are doing something about it.
- see yourself succeeding.
- value your mistakes. Learn from them. Do not judge them and do not judge or devalue yourself!

If procrastination is a habit of yours, forget it. Focus on the tasks and project at hand, and build from there.

Practicing Carefully.   Being responsible for the nursing care of others is a huge responsibility. To be successful, you must learn to perform your skills safely, in an approved manner. There is a reason for each step of the skill, even if the reason is not apparent to you. Avoid taking shortcuts. Learn, study, practice, and apply your skills in the manner that you learn in class. To be successful as a nursing assistant, you will need to commit the steps of these skills to memory so you can do them automatically. To do this, you must practice continually, in class and in your study group. Your instructor will plan skills laboratory and clinical activities to help you learn, develop, and master your skills. You have the responsibility to

■ seek experiences and skills you have been taught in the classroom and skills lab when you work in the clinical area. Inform your instructor or supervisor of skills you lack or those for which you need additional practice.

■ practice your skills under supervision until you and your instructor believe you can perform them safely and correctly. Make certain your instructor evaluates your performance and checks off the skills on your checklist before you do them on residents without direct supervision.

KEY POINTS

Developing a few basic study habits can be important to a lifetime of learning. A few simple steps will make learning easier and will help ensure success in your future study endeavors.

■ Be familiar with your text. This will save you time in finding information.

■ Master the steps to learning.

■ Practice becoming an active listener.

■ Take notes for reference and study.

■ Plan study times and practice in ways that promote learning.

■ Work on creating balance in your life.

■ Avoid procrastination.

ACTIVITIES

Vocabulary

Define the following terms in the spaces provided.

1. critical thinking _____

2. active listening _____

3. processing _____

4. procrastination _____

5. objectives _____

Completion

Complete the following statements by filling in the terms from the list provided.

10%	active listening	imprint
20%	carefully practicing and applying the information	key points
30%	critical thinking	processing
50%	distracts	
70%	effective studying	
90%		

6. The three basic steps to learning are _____, _____, and _____.

7. Daydreaming _____ you and interferes with your ability to listen actively.

8. The development of _____ skills should be a lifelong quest for health care workers.

9. Students remember _____% of what they read, _____% of what they hear, _____% of what they see, _____% of what they see and hear, _____% of what they say, and _____% of what they see and do together when performing an activity.

10. The _____ are a summary of important information presented in each chapter.

11. Taking notes is a good way to _____ what you are processing.

12. _____ involves making sense of new information in your brain.

13. As a nursing assistant, you can and will make a difference in the lives of many others. Rearrange the letters to form a sentence in the lower grid, and think of how this relates to you, your class, and your chosen career.

A	G		H		4		D		E	L	A		
T	U	I	T	E	R	A	E	0	E	S		M	I	O	W	S	E
B	O	T	F	L	A	V	N	D	T	H	E	S	P	C	E	T	R
B	U	T	L	E	Y	F	L	I	0	0	E	L	I	E	M	E	F	R

14. Follow the maze. Which path will you travel?

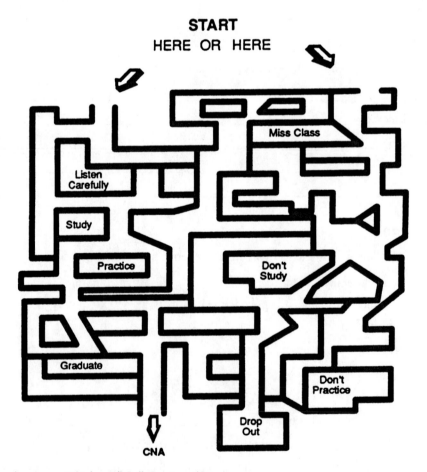

START
HERE OR HERE

FIGURE 5 Follow the maze. Which path will you travel?

PART I

Student Activities

CHAPTER 1

Introduction to Health Care

KEY POINTS

- Hospitals provide care to patients with acute illnesses.
- Long-term care facilities provide care to residents with chronic illnesses and those who need personal care.
- Subacute care is given to residents who have complex medical or rehabilitation needs.
- Skilled nursing facilities provide care to residents who are medically stable, but require daily skilled services and intervention by licensed health care professionals.
- Home care is provided to clients in their residences by qualified caregivers.
- The OBRA legislation was designed to improve the quality of life for residents of long-term care facilities. This legislation also specifies requirements for nursing assistant education.
- The health care agency, resident, nurse, and nursing assistant all benefit from nursing assistant education and certification.
- The nursing assistant is supervised by a licensed nurse.
- The interdisciplinary team is a group of caregivers who contribute to the care, health, and well-being of residents.
- The chain of command describes the lines of authority used in the health care facility for reporting information.
- Desirable qualities include a professional appearance, good personal hygiene and grooming, good personal health, responsible behavior, dependability, and good organizational skills.

ACTIVITIES

Vocabulary

Define the following terms in the spaces provided.

1. acute illness _____
2. attitude _____
3. care plan _____
4. chronic illness _____
5. client _____
6. dependable _____
7. empathy _____
8. hospice _____
9. hospital _____
10. immunization _____
11. interdisciplinary team _____
12. long-term care facilities _____

13. OBRA _____

14. patient _____

15. priorities _____

16. rehabilitation _____

17. resident _____

18. responsible behavior _____

19. restorative care _____

20. self-esteem _____

Fill in the Blanks

21. Federal law requires nursing assistants to complete at least _____ hours of continuing education every year to maintain certification.

22. The nursing assistant's immediate supervisor is a _____ _____.

23. The _____ _____ _____ is the line of authority that each department follows in reporting information.

24. _____ is the ability to say and do things at the right time.

25. _____ is emotional and physical tension that can be harmful to your health.

Short Answer

Complete the statements in the spaces provided.

26. List five requirements of the Omnibus Budget Reconciliation Act (OBRA).

_____

_____

_____

_____

_____

27. List five benefits of nursing assistant education to the individual, the residents, and/or the long-term care facility.

_____

_____

_____

_____

_____

28. List at least 10 members of the interdisciplinary team and state their responsibilities.

_____

_____

_____

_____

_____

_____

_____

_____

_____

_____

29. Explain why teamwork is important in health care facilities.

_____

_____

_____

_____

_____

30. List five ways to maintain your personal health and well-being.

_____

_____

_____

_____

_____

Completion

Fill in the blanks to complete the charts.

31. Identify positive and negative employee characteristics by placing an "X" in the proper column.

Characteristic	Positive	Negative
uniform clean and wrinkle-free		
long hair in face		
small post (stud) earrings		
long nails with bright, chipped nail polish		
uses antiperspirant		
clean, comfortable shoes		
rings on each finger		
multiple piercings in nose, tongue, etc.		
talking on cell phone from resident's room		
wears name (identification) badge		
doing tasks that need to be done without being asked		
calling in sick at least once a week		
not notifying the facility of an absence		
giving two weeks' notice of resignation		
helping other staff		
taking shortcuts to save time		
setting priorities and organizing time		
skipping continuing education classes		

32. Rearrange the letters to form a sentence in the lower grid. (Keep the letters in the same columns, skip a column for a space between words.)

				G	E	T		E	E		C	I			M		W	S	T			B	E			M			
T	H	E	T	O	E	T	E	A	L	N		E	O		L	I	S	I	E	L		T	N	I	T	G	E	N	R
K	S	I	G	I	N	T	T	H	I	I	V	T	N	D	A	F	N	A	N	T	L	I	E	A	I	H	W	I	T
S	H	T	O	H	A	S	T	R	D	R	S	A	L	P	O	S	A	I	R	Y	A	R	E	S	N	D	E	O	R

33. Complete the chart to list the proper lines of communication.

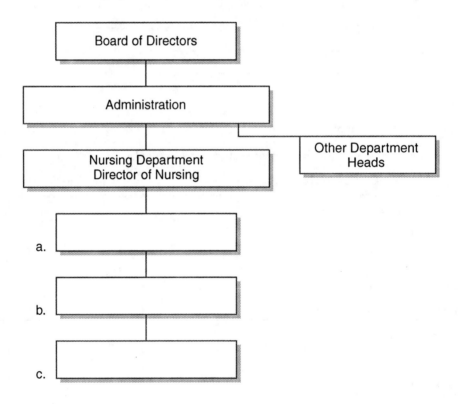

Developing Greater Insight

34. Maria is struggling to complete her assignment on time each day and is very frustrated. You realize she is not organizing her work or setting priorities. She asks you what she should do. What advice will you give her?

_____

_____

_____

_____

_____

35. Mrs. Sotolongo's family has complained that someone has been making long-distance calls on their mother's telephone. You have seen several different staff members using this phone when the resident was out of the room. What will you do?

_____

_____

_____

_____

_____

36. Mr. Decker is blind. He has had a stroke and cannot speak, although he seems to be alert. He listens to big-band music on the radio when he is in his room, and seems to enjoy it. When Cliff cares for the resident, he always changes the radio station to a hip-hop station. He sometimes forgets to change it back to the big-band station when he leaves the room. You can tell from the resident's facial expressions and body language that he does not like the hip-hop music. How will you handle this situation?

_____

_____

_____

_____

_____

37. Mrs. Paul is on a diabetic diet. She has had two sugar packets and other items, such as frosted cake, on her tray every night this week. You have switched them for the correct items, but the problem recurs again the next day. Using the chain of command, how will you handle this situation?

_____

_____

_____

_____

_____

38. Your name badge accidentally went through the washer and dryer and was ruined. You order another right away, but find it will take a week to get the new one. When you go to work without a name badge, you realize that a resident's family thinks you are a nurse. What will you do?

_____

_____

_____

_____

_____

39. One of your children is acting up and upsetting you at home. Things have been busier than usual at work. You feel very frustrated, and realize you have been short with residents and coworkers. What will you do?

_____

_____

_____

_____

_____

40. There are two new residents in room 403. One is on a low-salt diet and the other is on a diabetic diet. After dinner, you realize you have accidentally switched their meal trays. The residents are sitting up visiting, and there are no visible harmful effects. What will you do?

_____

_____

_____

_____

_____

CHAPTER 2

Working in Long-Term Care

KEY POINTS

- Quality of life is very important for residents of a long-term care facility.

- Residents in long-term care facilities are like you in many ways.

- Aging affects the function of the entire body.

- All human beings have the same basic needs, which are described in Maslow's hierarchy of needs.

- The OBRA legislation states that declines in residents' condition are not permitted unless they are medically unavoidable.

- It is important to look at the resident holistically. View the resident as a complex person with many strengths and needs.

- Basic resident care skills include providing personal care, providing food service and mealtime assistance, observation and reporting, caring for the resident's unit and belongings, caring for equipment and supplies, recordkeeping, and messenger duties.

- Developing good relationships with residents is important.

- Professional boundaries are unspoken limits on physical and emotional relationships that limit and define how a health care worker acts. Respecting boundaries involves using your best behavior, ethical practices, and good judgment when caring for residents.

ACTIVITIES

Vocabulary

Using the definitions provided, unscramble the words. Put the appropriate numbers in the blanks below.

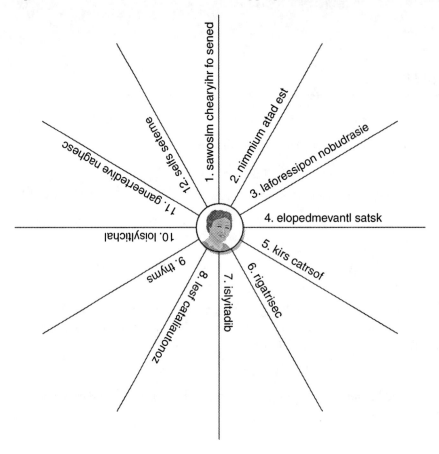

1. _____ A chart based on a widely accepted theory of physical and psychological needs of all human beings.

2. _____ The assessment tool upon which the care plan is based; completed upon admission and quarterly for all residents of long-term care facilities.

3. _____ Unspoken limits on physical and emotional relationships that limit and define how a health care worker acts.

4. _____ Intellectual, social, and emotional skills that a person must accomplish at a certain age.

5. _____ Conditions that have the potential to cause the resident's health to worsen or indicate that a problem may develop.

6. _____ Care of the elderly.

7. _____ Inability to function normally because of a physical or mental problem.

8. _____ The realization of one's full potential.

9. _____ Commonly accepted beliefs that have no basis in fact.

10. _____ Viewing the resident as a whole person with many complex strengths and needs.

11. _____ Deterioration of a body part or system due to age or disease.

12. _____ Your opinion of yourself.

Completion

13. Complete the table in the spaces provided.

System	Function	Organs
Nervous		brain, spinal cord, nerves
	Transports, digests, absorbs nutrients from food, eliminates waste	mouth, teeth, tongue, salivary glands, pharynx, esophagus, liver, gallbladder, stomach, small intestine, large intestine, appendix, rectum, anus
Urinary	Regulation of fluid balance, elimination of liquid waste	
Endocrine		Pituitary gland, pineal gland, parathyroid gland, thyroid gland, adrenal glands, thymus glands, testes, ovaries
Circulatory	Carries and transports oxygen and water to body and eliminates waste	
	Protects against infection, removes waste, sensory perception	Nails, sweat and oil glands, hair, skin
Skeletal		Bones, joints
Reproductive		Female: uterus, fallopian tubes, ovaries. Male: penis, prostate, testes, scrotum.
Respiratory	Supplies oxygen and eliminates carbon dioxide	
	Allows movement of body	Muscles, ligaments, tendons

Complete the following statements by filling in the terms from the list provided.

anus	declines	esophagus	kidneys	trachea
arteries	dermis	fecal material	larynx	urethra
bladder	epidermis	insulin	risk factors	veins

14. The thinner, outer layer of the skin is the _____.

15. The _____ is a hollow muscle in which urine is stored until it is eliminated from the body.

16. _____ is solid waste eliminated from the digestive system.

17. The _____ are the organs that filter waste products from the blood and produce urine.

18. The _____ is the thicker, inner layer of the skin.

19. The _____ is the voice box.

20. _____ are a worsening or deterioration in the resident's physical or mental condition.

21. The _____ is the upper windpipe extending from the larynx to the bronchus.

22. The _____ is the outlet of the intestines at the rectum, from which waste products are eliminated.

23. The _____ is the hollow tube leading from the bladder to the outside of the body.

24. The _____ is the tube through which food passes from the back of the throat to the stomach.

25. _____ is a hormone secreted by the pancreas that regulates glucose metabolism.

26. _____ are blood vessels that carry blood from the body parts back to the heart.

27. _____ are conditions that have the potential to cause the resident's health to worsen or indicate that problems may develop.

28. The _____ are blood vessels that carry freshly oxygenated blood to nourish body parts.

True/False

Mark the following statements true or false.

29. T   F   Similar tissues form larger structures called organs.

30. T   F   The human body has 10 systems.

31. T   F   Hemiparesis is weakness on one side of the body.

32. T   F   Paraplegia is paralysis of the arms and legs.

33. T   F   Signs and symptoms of TIA are similar to those of a stroke, but are reversible and temporary.

34. T   F   Young and middle-aged residents of a facility often view staff as their peer group.

35. T   F   The nursing assistant's personal goal should be to contribute to providing the highest quality of life possible for each resident.

36. T   F   Nursing assistants are encouraged to become close friends with the residents.

37. T   F   To provide consistency of care, nursing assistants should control residents' routines as much as possible.

38. T   F   Caregivers may not recognize unhealthy relationships until it is too late.

39. T   F   Most nursing assistants are immune from having unhealthy relationships with residents.

40. T   F   Boundary violations may cause workers to do things they would not ordinarily do, such as stealing from the employer.

41. T   F   The immune system is the part of the circulatory system that recognizes foreign germs in the body and helps fight disease.

42. T   F   The reproductive system plays a major role in maintaining fluid balance in the body.

43. T   F   Enlargement of the prostate gland is a common aging change.

44. T   F   Food moves through the intestines more rapidly in young adults than it does in the elderly.

45. T   F   Healthy elderly individuals are at no greater risk of injury than younger adults.

46. T   F   Dryness and itching are normal aging changes that occur to the eyes.

47. T   F   Mental confusion is a normal aging change that occurs as a result of brain shrinkage.

48. T   F   Loss of bowel and bladder control are normal aging changes.

49. T   F   The skeletal system contributes to the production of blood cells and calcium storage.

50. T   F   The muscular system helps produce heat in the body.

51. T   F   As we age, the heart weakens, causing blood vessels to become more fragile and break more easily.

52. T   F   Senile purpura are purple bruises that commonly develop in the elderly as a result of minor injuries.

53. T   F   Skin tears are uncommon in elderly adults.

54. T   F   Skin tears are irregular-shaped injuries in which the top layer of the skin peels back.

55. T   F   Blood supply to the feet and legs decreases with age, increasing the risk of serious injury.
56. T   F   Diabetes is a chronic illness that affects the utilization of sugar in the body in about 10% of adults over the age of 65.
57. T   F   Elderly persons can enjoy an active sex life.
58. T   F   When needs on a lower level of Maslow's hierarchy of needs are not met, residents will experience physical problems.
59. T   F   Needs at the higher levels of Maslow's hierarchy of needs are essential for survival.
60. T   F   Developmental tasks become more complex as a person grows and ages.

Identification

61. Identify the structure of the human body by filling in each circle.

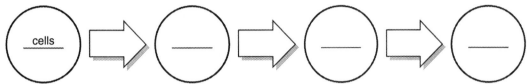

62. Identify the four basic types of tissues in the human body and state their purpose.

_____

_____

_____

_____

Identify declines by writing a D on the line. Identify normal aging changes or problems caused by a disease process by writing an N on the line.

63. _____ A resident developed two Stage II pressure ulcers yesterday.
64. _____ Mrs. Eagger says she is constipated at least once a week.
65. _____ Mr. DelPecchio had bowel and bladder control on admission, but became incontinent within a few weeks.
66. _____ Miss Love is overweight and is often seen eating candy. She was discovered to have elevated blood sugar. The nurse said they are testing her for diabetes.
67. _____ Mr. Luna's care plan says to dress him in a long-sleeved shirt to protect his arms. Susan dressed him in a t-shirt, and he got a skin tear.
68. _____ Mrs. Washington has dry, itchy eyes.
69. _____ Mr. Tinsley has an open area on his toe from his shoe rubbing against it.
70. _____ Three residents on B wing have a urinary infection caused by the same organism.
71. _____ The doctor said Mr. McKay's Alzheimer's disease is worsening.
72. _____ Mr. Hillyer is at high risk of blood clots if his legs are injured.
73. _____ Mrs. Hernandez has arthritic pain in her hands.
74. _____ Mr. Lake needs stronger glasses.
75. _____ Susan Munden had hip replacement surgery and returned from the hospital with a red area on her left heel. The nurse said it was a Stage I pressure ulcer, and wrote a care plan to elevate the heels. Within two days, the area on the left heel was a Stage IV pressure ulcer, and the right heel had a Stage I area.

76. _____ Miss Kaiser just had a urinalysis, which was normal. She wakes up to urinate every two hours during the night.

Matching

Match the organs with the proper system.

77. _____ adrenal gland

78. _____ alveoli

79. _____ urethra

80. _____ brain

81. _____ transverse colon

82. _____ arteries

83. _____ achilles tendon

84. _____ femur

85. _____ uterus

86. _____ skin

a. cardiovascular (circulatory)

b. respiratory

c. gastrointestinal (digestive)

d. urinary

e. endocrine

f. reproductive

g. skeletal

h. muscular

i. integumentary

j. nervous

Labeling

Label the following diagrams.

87.

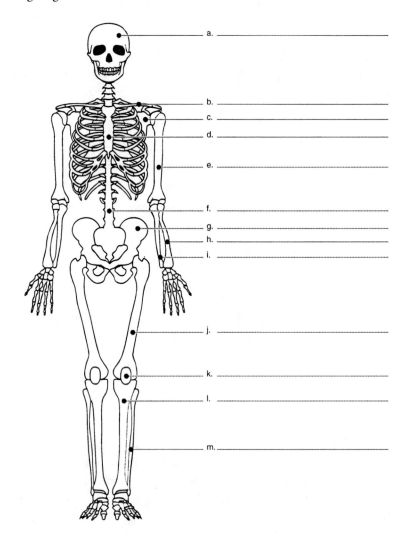

a. _____

b. _____

c. _____

d. _____

e. _____

f. _____

g. _____

h. _____

i. _____

j. _____

k. _____

l. _____

m. _____

88.

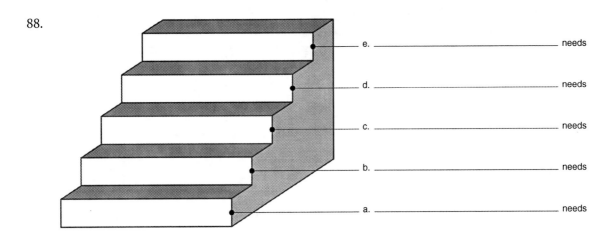

e. _____ needs

d. _____ needs

c. _____ needs

b. _____ needs

a. _____ needs

Developing Greater Insight

89. Mrs. Hoyle does not want to get out of bed. She says she does not want a bath right now. During the conversation, she shows you an old photograph of a beautiful young woman, and says it is a picture of her when she was a professional model. She confides that she feels so old and ugly that she doesn't want anyone to see her. How can you assist this resident?

_____

_____

_____

_____

_____

90. Mrs. Hernandez has a care plan that notes she is at very high risk of skin injury. The plan lists approaches to prevent injuries, such as bruises, skin tears, and pressure ulcers. Why is it important to identify the resident's high-risk conditions?

_____

_____

_____

_____

_____

CHAPTER 3

Infection Control

KEY POINTS

- Medical asepsis refers to practices used in health care facilities to prevent the spread of infection.

- Microorganisms are everywhere. Pathogens are microorganisms that cause disease.

- The most common methods of spreading infection are airborne, droplet, direct contact, and indirect contact.

- The nursing assistant plays an important role in preventing the spread of infection.

- The nursing assistant must know which items are considered clean and which are considered soiled. These items must be separated to prevent the spread of infection.

- Handwashing is the most important method used to prevent the spread of infection.

- Bloodborne pathogens are microbes that cause disease through contact with blood, any moist body fluid except sweat, secretions, excretions, nonintact skin, and mucous membranes.

- HIV disease, hepatitis B, and hepatitis C are examples of diseases that are spread by contact with bloodborne pathogens.

- Hepatitis B is a greater threat to health care workers than HIV.

- Standard precautions are measures used in the care of all residents to prevent the spread of disease.

- The nursing assistant is responsible for selecting and using the correct personal protective equipment for the procedure being performed.

- Needles, razors, and other sharps are disposed of in puncture-resistant biohazardous waste containers.

- Trash or linen that have contacted blood or body fluids are biohazardous waste.

- Isolation can be emotionally difficult for the resident.

- A HEPA mask is used when a resident is in airborne precautions. A PFR95, N95, or other NIOSH-approved respirator may be worn instead.

- A surgical mask is worn when a resident is in droplet precautions.

- A gown and gloves are used when a resident is in contact precautions.

- Standard precautions are used in addition to transmission-based precautions.

- Transmission-based precautions are isolation categories designed to interrupt the mode of transmission so the pathogen cannot spread.

- Drug-resistant organisms are a problem in health care facilities. Their spread can be prevented by medical asepsis and use of standard precautions.

- Tuberculosis is a growing public health problem that is detected by a skin test and treated with antibiotics.

- Head lice and scabies are highly contagious and require the use of contact precautions for 24 hours after the resident is treated.

- *Escherichia coli* is a type of bacteria that normally resides in the intestines. It can cause serious illness outside the intestinal tract.

- *E. coli 0157:H7* is a nonhuman strain that is found in the intestines of some cattle. It is most commonly spread in undercooked hamburger, and has caused outbreaks resulting in serious illness and death.

- Pseudomembranous colitis occurs when antibiotics destroy the normal, helpful bowel flora, except for *C. difficile*. Without the other friendly bacteria to keep it in check, it breeds rapidly, producing toxins that cause diarrhea and serious illness.

- Hantavirus causes serious respiratory illness. It is spread by contact with rodents or their excretions, including urine and stool.

- Shingles develop only in individuals who have had chickenpox. The resident develops painful, blister-like lesions on the torso that are often mistaken for a rash.

- Health care workers who have not had chickenpox should not enter the room of a resident with shingles, if other immune caregivers are available.

- Bioterrorism is the use of biological agents, such as pathogenic organisms or agricultural pests, for terrorist purposes.

ACTIVITIES

Vocabulary

1. Complete the crossword puzzle.

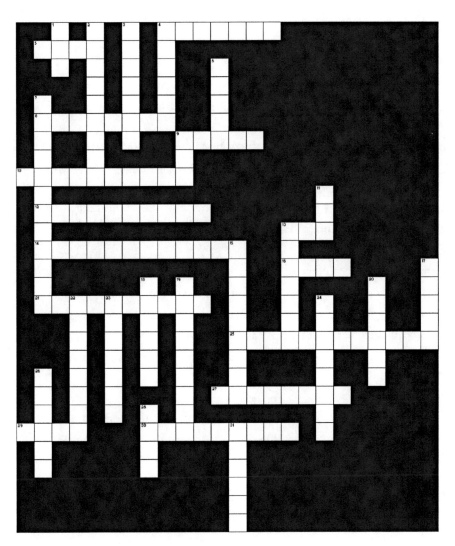

Across

4 In the _____ method of transmission, pathogens are spread by secretions produced when laughing, talking, singing, sneezing, or coughing.

5 a tiny parasite that cannot be seen with the eye; the causative agent for scabies

8 _____ contact involves touching objects, equipment, linens, environmental surfaces, trash, or dishes contaminated with harmful pathogens.

9 A description of the factors necessary for an infection to spread. If one link in the _____ is broken, an infection cannot be spread.

10 chemical agent used for cleansing the skin

12 Human waste products eliminated from the body

13 vancomycin-resistant Enterococcus

14 The mode of _____ is the method by which a pathogen is spread.

16 the place where a disease-causing germ can grow

21 A _____ infection develops in a health care facility.

25 a contagious disease spread by the airborne method; it commonly affects the lungs, but can cause illness in other parts of the body

27 Apply the principles of _____ precautions in all resident care.

29 acquired immune deficiency syndrome

30 Living or nonliving material in or on which a pathogen lives and multiplies. The pathogen is dependent on this host for its survival.

Down

1 human immunodeficiency virus, the pathogen that causes HIV disease and AIDS

2 inflammation of the liver caused by a number of factors, including drugs, toxins, autoimmune disease, and infectious agents

3 A person who can give a disease to others; he or she may not know of the infection.

4 _____ contact involves the spread of infection by touching.

6 Normal _____ are microbes that are healthy and necessary for the body to function correctly; they are not harmful in the area in which they reside, but can cause infection if they spread to other parts of the body.

7 a chemical cleaning process that destroys most microbes; usually used to clean reusable items

9 Centers for Disease Control

11 personal protective equipment

13 food, water, medication, or another substance taken into the body in which pathogens can live and multiply

15 Having _____ skin that is broken, cut, chapped, or cracked increases the risk of infection.

17 A tiny pathogen that causes disease; antibiotics will not eliminate it.

18 The _____ system is a part of the circulatory system that recognizes invading germs and works to eliminate them from the body.

19 disease-causing microbes

20 _____ membranes are body tissues that secrete mucus; these areas open to the outside of the body and are very susceptible to the spread of infection.

22 A condition that develops in people who have had chickenpox. Painful, blister-like lesions that follow the nerve pathways appear on the torso.

23 A resident with a skin infection will be placed in _____ precautions.

24 one-celled microorganisms that can cause disease

26   an environmental surface, supplies, linen, or equipment contaminated with pathogens

28   methicillin-resistant staphylococcus aureus

31   an insect, rodent, or small animal that spreads disease

Matching

Match the terms and description.

Description

  2. _____ tiny pathogens suspended in dust and moisture in the air that are inhaled by the susceptible host

  3. _____ the ability of the body to resist disease

  4. _____ medications that eliminate pathogens from the body

  5. _____ drainage, discharge, or seeping from the body

  6. _____ a state of sickness or disease caused by pathogens in the body

  7. _____ living germs that cannot be seen with the eye

  8. _____ tiny animals that survive by feeding off another human or animal

  9. _____ mucus and secretions containing a pathogen from oral, nasal, and respiratory secretions

10. _____ spread throughout the entire body

11. _____ a virus that is spread by contact with rodents (rats and mice) or their excretions, including urine and stool

12. _____ measures used when a resident has an infectious disease; prevents the spread of pathogens to others

13. _____ a skin condition caused by a mite; it causes a rash and severe itching and is highly contagious

14. _____ a yellow skin color caused by hepatitis and some other diseases

15. _____ the use of biological agents, such as pathogenic organisms or agricultural pests, for terrorist purposes

16. _____ confined to a specific area of the body

17. _____ microbes that cause diseases spread through contact with blood or body fluid

18. _____ disposable items that are contaminated with blood or body fluids

19. _____ the way in which an infection is spread

20. _____ touching objects, equipment, or other materials contaminated with pathogens

21. _____ small purplish spots on the body surface, caused by minute hemorrhage

22. _____ an enlarged abdomen

Terms

a.   hantavirus

b.   droplets

c.   isolation

d.   microorganisms

e.   indirect contact

f.   petechia

g.   antibiotics

h.   generalized

i.   distended

j.   bloodborne pathogens

k.   airborne

l.   mode of transmission

m.   secretions

n.   biohazardous waste

o.   jaundice

p.   localized

q.   parasites

r.   susceptibility

s.   bioterrorism

t.   infection

u.   scabies

Completion

Write the information in the space provided.

23. Complete the chain of infection.

    a. _____

    b. _____

    c. _____

    d. _____

    e. _____

24. List three ways to break the chain of infection.

    a. _____

    b. _____

    c. _____

25. What happens if a link in the chain of infection is broken?

_____

26. List three ways in which pathogens are spread.

    a. _____

    b. _____

    c. _____

27. List 10 ways to prevent the spread of infection.

    a. _____

    b. _____

    c. _____

    d. _____

    e. _____

    f. _____

    g. _____

    h. _____

    i. _____

    j. _____

28. Liquid soap should be used whenever possible. Explain why bar soap should not be used.

_____

_____

29. List at least fifteen times when handwashing should be done.

    a. _____

    b. _____

    c. _____

    d. _____

    e. _____

f. _____

g. _____

h. _____

i. _____

j. _____

k. _____

l. _____

m. _____

n. _____

o. _____

30. Identify times when alcohol-based, waterless hand cleaner may be used with an "A" (for alcohol). Identify times when handwashing should be done at the sink with an "S" (for sink).

a. when entering the room to give resident care _____

b. after feeding a resident and getting food on your hand _____

c. after touching an unidentified moist, sticky substance on the countertop _____

d. before applying gloves to assist with a bedpan _____

e. after removing gloves used for assisting with a urinal _____

f. when hands are dusty after moving boxes of supplies _____

31. List five ways in which bloodborne pathogens are spread.

a. _____

b. _____

c. _____

d. _____

e. _____

32. Identify the personal protective equipment to use for each of the following tasks by placing an "X" in the proper column.

Task	None	Gloves	Gown	Mask	Face Shield or Goggles
Shaving a resident with a disposable razor					
Changing a bed that is heavily soiled with diarrhea stool					
Changing a bed in which the linen is not visibly soiled					
Emptying a very full catheter bag that is splashing					
Removing a urinal					
Washing a resident's arms and legs when skin is intact					

Task	None	Gloves	Gown	Mask	Face Shield or Goggles
Assisting the nurse while he suctions a resident who is coughing and spitting up secretions					
Brushing a resident's dentures					
Combing a resident's hair that is long and tangled					
Assisting a resident with persistent vomiting					

33. Identify the personal protective equipment to use for each of the following tasks for a resident who is in isolation by placing an "X" in the proper column.

Task	Type of Isolation	Gloves	Gown	Surgical Mask	HEPA Mask	Face Shield or Goggles
Answering the call signal	Airborne					
Serving a meal tray	Contact					
Changing a bed in which the linen is not visibly soiled	Contact					
Serving a meal tray	Droplet					
Removing a urinal	Droplet					
Serving a meal tray	Airborne					
Removing a bedpan	Airborne					
Giving a shower	Contact					
Assisting the dentist with a confused resident who is coughing	Contact					
Changing a bed in which the resident has vomited on the linen	Contact					

34. List the order in which to apply gown, gloves, mask, and face shield.

_____

35. List the order in which to remove gown, gloves, mask, and face shield.

_____

True/False

Mark the following statements true or false.

36. T   F   Medical asepsis is also called infection control.

37. T   F   People who are HIV positive have AIDS.

38. T   F   People with hepatitis C are lifelong carriers of the disease.

39. T   F   Hepatitis B can be cured if diagnosed early.

40. T   F   The biohazard emblem is black with an orange symbol.

41. T   F   Drug resistance is a very serious problem.

42. T   F   Night sweats, feeling tired, and shortness of breath are signs and symptoms of tuberculosis.

43. T   F   A resident with scabies is placed in droplet precautions.

44. T   F   Head lice hop and fly from one person to another.

45. T   F   Isolation categories are designed to interrupt the mode of transmission.

46. T   F   Escherichia coli 0157:H7 is transmitted by direct contact.

47. T   F   Pseudomembranous colitis is a very serious condition in which diarrhea is caused by *Clostridium difficile.*

48. T   F   *Clostridium difficile* can reside on bedpans, bedside commodes, toilets, sinks, countertops, bed rails, doorknobs, and other surfaces that have been contaminated by stool.

49. T   F   Hantavirus is spread by ticks.

50. T   F   Shingles blisters are not contagious.

51. T   F   Caregivers who have not had chickenpox should not care for residents with shingles.

52. T   F   Artificial nails may be worn at work, but should not extend more than half an inch from the fingertips.

53. T   F   Many infections are spread on the hands.

54. T   F   Petechiae are large bruises commonly seen in residents with MRSA.

55. T   F   Microbes may hide under finger rings.

56. T   F   Tuberculosis is spread by the droplet method.

57. T   F   Scabies are not very contagious.

Identification

Identify the sign and indicate the type of precautions used.

58. a. _____   _____

    b. _____   _____

    c. _____   _____

    d. _____   _____

    e. _____   _____

Developing Greater Insight

59. You must select personal protective equipment to care for Mrs. Martin, a resident who has had diarrhea. Her pants are soiled, and the stool has run into her shoes. The nurse instructs you to give the resident a shower. What protective equipment will you wear? Who are you protecting when you wear PPE?

   _____

   _____

   _____

CHAPTER 4

Safety and Emergencies

KEY POINTS

- Every employee of the health care facility is responsible for keeping the environment safe.

- Changes in vision, hearing, blood vessels, and reflexes put some residents at high risk for accidents.

- You should correct unsafe conditions, if possible, or report them to the proper person.

- Material safety data sheets give instructions for safe use of chemicals, identify health risks of chemicals, and describe first aid and safety precautions.

- You should answer the call lights of all residents, whether you are assigned to care for the resident or not.

- Identify the resident before giving care.

- Before applying a heat or cold application, know the type of application, area to be treated, length of time the application is to be used, proper temperature, safety precautions, and side effects to watch for.

- The nursing assistant must know and practice oxygen safety.

- Oxygen, fuel, and a spark are necessary to start a fire.

- In a fire emergency, the RACE system is used to remove residents from danger, activate the alarm, contain, and extinguish the fire.

- Know and follow facility policies for tornado, hurricane, earthquake, and bomb threat emergencies.

- The Occupational Safety and Health Administration is an agency that is responsible for overseeing employee safety in the workplace.

- If you discover a resident who is having a medical emergency or is injured, stay with the resident and call for help.

- The universal sign for choking is one or both hands on the throat.

- The speed with which defibrillation is performed is the key to success in cardiac arrest. In the community, defibrillation within five minutes is a goal; in health care facilities, defibrillation within three minutes is the goal.

ACTIVITIES

Vocabulary

Each line has four different spellings of a word from this unit. Circle the correctly spelled word.

1.	occedents	accidents	axidens	accydints
2.	asspiration	aspration	assprashun	aspiration
3.	ora	orruh	aura	orea
4.	chemicals	kemicals	chemichaels	khemicals
5.	cunstricts	cunstricks	constricts	contricts
6.	eckynoses	ecchymosis	eckymoses	eshkymosis
7.	dinial	denaisle	dinysle	denial
8.	dielate	dialate	dilate	dylate
9.	eddema	idema	edema	aedema
10.	epiglottis	eppiglotis	ipiglottis	epiglottes
11.	fackshual	factual	facshall	factaull
12.	flammible	flameabl	fameble	flammable
13.	generalized	genralized	generelised	gennralised
14.	hemorage	hemerage	hemorrhage	hemrage
15.	humidifyer	humiddefyer	humydifire	humidifier
16.	identification	idenificashun	identyfication	idenification
17.	imobilize	immobylize	immobilize	imobilise
18.	incedent	insidant	insident	incident
19.	loculized	localized	localised	loccelized
20.	obstructed	ubstructed	obstruced	ubstracted
21.	reflecces	reflexes	reaflaxes	reflecis
22.	ressolved	risolved	rissolfed	resolved
23.	seasshore	seesure	seizure	siezurr
24.	shock	chock	shoke	shoek
25.	sincopee	sincupe	syncope	sinncope
26.	tepped	teped	tiped	tepid
27.	thurmel	thirmul	thermal	thermul
28.	tornado	tornadoe	tornato	tornadow
29.	tremmors	tremors	tremirs	tremurs
30.	chocking	chokeng	showking	choking
31.	vitle	vitale	vital	vitull

Completion

Complete the statements regarding safety practices by selecting the correct term from the list.

72 hours	checked	hands	OSHA	smoking
after shave	container	heat	oxygen	spark
alcohol	electrical	incident	perfume	stay with the resident
all health care	elevator	Legionnaire's disease	reach	wrist
base	footwear	locked	residents	upright
burns	fuel	MSDS	right away	tagged
calm	grounded	never		

32. Keeping the environment safe and clean is the responsibility of _____ workers.

33. The call light should always be within the resident's _____.

34. Wheels should always be _____ unless a bed is being moved.

35. Frayed _____ cords should be reported at once.

36. Never pick up broken glass with your _____.

37. An unexpected, undesirable event that occurs in a health care facility is an _____.

38. When equipment is broken, it is _____.

39. Electrical and mechanical equipment should be _____ before use.

40. Plugs that are not properly _____ are a fire hazard.

41. Smoking in bed should _____ be permitted.

42. The three elements that form the fire triangle are _____, _____, and _____.

43. Possible fire hazards should be reported to the supervisor _____

44. When oxygen is used, flammable liquids such as _____, _____, or _____ should not be used.

45. A fire extinguisher should be carried in the _____ position.

46. Remain _____ in an emergency.

47. In a fire, move _____ to safety first.

48. The federal agency responsible for worker safety is _____.

49. Hazard communication called _____ must be supplied by manufacturers.

50. Aim the fire extinguisher at the _____ of the fire.

51. Make sure _____ is appropriate for the floor surface.

52. If a thermometer is not available, check water temperature on the inside of your _____.

53. Never use the _____ in a fire emergency.

54. Complications of head injuries may not be apparent until _____ or longer after the injury.

55. In an emergency, _____ and call for help.

56. Liquid oxygen will cause severe _____ upon direct contact.

57. If you suspect that a resident has swallowed a chemical, take the _____ to the nurse immediately.

58. Inhalation of tap water is associated with _____.

59. _____ applications dilate blood vessels.

60. Careless and unsupervised _____ is a major cause of fire in long term care facilities.

Completion

Write the information in the space provided.

61. These acronyms are important for fire control. The

    a. P stands for _____ .   e. R stands for _____ .

    b. A stands for _____ .   f. A stands for _____ .

    c. S stands for _____ .   g. C stands for _____ .

    d. S stands for _____ .   h. E stands for _____ .

62. The MSDS provides information on _____

_____

63. Two types of heat and cold applications are _____ and _____ .

64. Heat and cold applications should always be _____ to prevent injury to the resident's skin.

65. The Aquamatic K-pad control unit should be filled with _____ .

66. The metal cap on an ice bag should always be positioned _____ from the resident.

67. Before using a heat or cold application, you should know the

    a. _____

    b. _____

    c. _____

    d. _____

    e. _____

    f. _____

68. An oxygen _____ should not be used in an emergency.

69. An oxygen mask should not be used if the liter flow is below _____ .

70. When selecting a fire extinguisher, the

    a. A is used for _____

    b. B is used for _____

    c. C is used for _____

    d. ABC is used for _____

71. You are in a resident's room when the fire alarm sounds. You should _____ .

72. When you touch the door, it is hot. You should _____ .

73. When caring for a resident who is having a seizure, your goal should be to _____ .

74. A resident has fallen. You suspect a hip fracture because one leg is _____ and _____ .

75. _____ burns are caused by flame and hot objects.

76. _____ burns are caused by harmful substances contacting the skin, eyes, or mucous membranes.

77. When caring for a resident who is bleeding, you should apply the principles of _____ .

78. When an unconscious resident is vomiting, you should _____ to prevent _____ .

79. Placing one or both hands on the throat is the _____ , which indicates that the person is _____ .

80. If you see someone with the hands at the throat, the first thing you should do is _____ .

81. When doing abdominal thrusts, avoid squeezing on the _____ with your forearms.

82. List six potential ways of preventing violence in the health care facility.

    a. _____

    b. _____

    c. _____

    d. _____

    e. _____

    f. _____

83. List six methods of dealing with a violent individual.

    a. _____

    b. _____

    c. _____

    d. _____

    e. _____

    f. _____

84. Draw the fire triangle. Label each element.

    a. _____

    b. _____

    c. _____

Hidden Picture

Look closely at the picture below. List each safety violation on 85 to 98 on the next page.

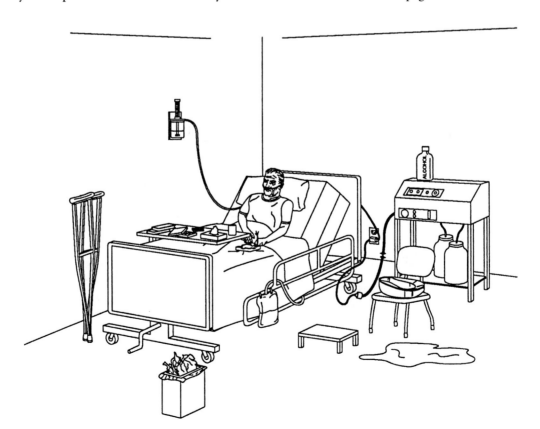

85. _____

86. _____

87. _____

88. _____

89. _____

90. _____

91. _____

92. _____

93. _____

94. _____

95. _____

96. _____

97. _____

98. _____

Developing Greater Insight

99. Mrs. Kreiter has a sprained ankle that is swollen and very painful. The ice pack keeps falling off. The resident puts on the call signal each time, and you replace the pack only to have the problem recur. What can the nursing assistant do to keep the ice pack in place?

    _____

100. The nursing assistant left a pitcher of hot water at the bedside so she could warm Mr. Lowe's foot soak. Mr. Lowe is confused. You hear him yell and enter the room to find he has poured the water all over himself. He has red areas that appear to be burned. What action will you take?

    _____

101. Rearrange the letters to form a sentence in the lower grid. (Keep the letters in the same columns; skip a column for a space between words.)

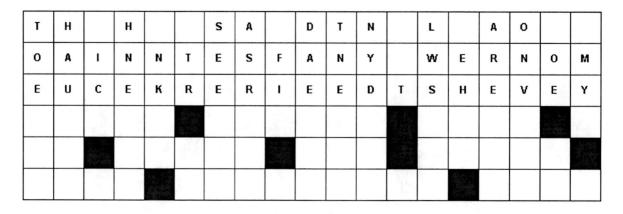

CHAPTER 5

Legal and Ethical Responsibilities

KEY POINTS

- Residents in long-term care facilities have specific legal rights that are guaranteed by the federal government.
- Nursing assistants must respect and protect the residents' rights. If the residents are unable to exercise these rights, the nursing assistant should assist.
- Professional boundaries are limits on how a health care worker acts with residents.
- The resident's culture and religion influence your ability to provide care.
- Restorative care is given to assist the resident to attain and maintain the highest level of independence possible.

ACTIVITIES

Vocabulary

Find and circle the words in the following puzzle. In phrases, only the words in italics are hidden in the puzzle. Define each word or phrase.

1. abandonment _____
2. abuse _____
3. *advance directive* _____
4. confidentiality _____
5. consent _____
6. cultures _____
7. *defamation* of character _____
8. *durable power* of *attorney* for health care _____
9. false *imprisonment* _____
10. *Good Samaritan* laws _____
11. grievance _____
12. health care *proxy* _____
13. *involuntary seclusion* _____
14. libel _____
15. *living will* _____
16. malpractice _____
17. *misappropriation* of property _____
18. neglect _____
19. negligence _____
20. ombudsman _____

21. personal *space* _____

22. *reasonable accommodation* _____

23. reprisal _____

24. Resident's Bill of *Rights* _____

25. *restorative* care _____

26. slander _____

27. *standards* of care _____

28. stereotyping _____

c	e	m	R	l	s	p	a	c	e	X	k	y	K	r	c	c	n	Z	a	S	r
d	u	c	i	i	e	z	R	c	G	Q	h	N	e	o	o	e	g	t	v	U	e
e	p	l	n	s	g	b	J	C	S	C	v	s	n	n	g	n	t	H	q	Y	s
f	r	c	t	a	a	h	i	V	S	f	u	f	s	l	i	o	t	l	v	L	t
a	o	M	d	u	v	p	t	l	e	b	i	e	e	v	r	f	v	G	F	e	o
m	x	D	H	V	r	d	p	s	a	d	n	c	i	n	s	a	f	B	T	c	r
a	y	j	V	l	v	e	a	r	e	t	t	l	e	m	t	y	X	I	T	n	a
t	B	a	v	J	a	b	s	n	o	g	S	y	M	T	A	Q	f	B	C	e	t
i	a	t	O	e	c	k	t	e	n	p	r	a	s	Y	i	i	U	d	r	g	i
o	G	U	V	f	a	i	v	n	d	o	r	i	m	d	r	e	O	n	e	i	v
n	A	X	r	a	a	i	a	n	p	u	i	i	e	a	r	e	n	b	w	l	e
C	c	E	U	l	t	m	o	L	w	p	r	t	a	v	r	a	d	G	o	g	g
a	b	v	i	c	s	i	l	c	w	i	x	a	a	t	a	i	d	n	p	e	Q
Z	r	t	e	d	s	a	k	v	a	b	X	q	b	d	i	n	t	n	a	n	l
y	y	r	u	u	s	P	R	G	T	E	l	e	t	l	o	o	c	a	a	l	Y
K	i	b	l	i	M	g	x	b	O	C	d	o	o	G	e	m	n	e	n	t	s
d	m	c	r	r	e	a	s	o	n	a	b	l	e	X	G	G	m	f	Z	i	s
o	e	p	w	p	s	k	e	c	i	t	c	a	r	p	l	a	m	o	P	O	Y
s	e	i	n	v	o	l	u	n	t	a	r	y	M	Q	B	N	z	z	c	b	g
r	s	C	n	S	R	f	E	r	t	n	e	m	n	o	d	n	a	b	a	c	U
s	t	e	r	e	o	t	y	p	i	n	g	l	P	i	W	b	l	G	Z	R	a
p	e	c	Y	a	X	l	C	i	w	t	n	e	m	n	o	s	i	r	p	m	i

Completion

Complete the following statements by selecting the correct term from the list provided here.

ability	federal	Residents' Bill of Rights
ask	illegal	safe
business	infringe	standard of care
confidentiality	policies	
explain	procedures	

29. The Omnibus Budget Reconciliation Act of 1987 is a _____ law.

30. A copy of the _____ is given to the resident upon admission to the long-term care facility.

31. Residents have the right to _____ in their personal information and health care records.

32. Facilities have _____ and _____ governing employee conduct and resident care.

33. Residents have a right to _____ care.

34. Residents may not _____ on the rights of others.

35. Abuse and neglect are _____.

36. Negligence involves breaching the _____.

37. Nursing assistants should not discuss facility _____ with others who are not employed by the facility.

38. The best way to find out about personal and cultural preferences is to _____ the resident.

39. The nursing assistant should always _____ procedures to residents before doing them.

40. Always stress the residents' _____ and not the disability.

Completion

Place an X in the box to determine what action has taken place.

Action	Neglect	Physical Abuse	Mental Abuse	Verbal Abuse	Sexual Abuse
41. Using an obscene gesture					
42. Calling a resident a demeaning name, such as "you pig"					
43. Failing to provide incontinent care, leaving a resident wet or soiled for a long time					
44. Hitting a resident					
45. Failing to turn a resident every two hours, as stated on the care plan					
46. Touching a resident in a sexual manner					
47. Forgetting to feed a resident					
48. Telling a resident that if he does not get dressed, he will not get his lunch.					
49. Jerking the resident out of the bed and throwing him down into the chair during a transfer					
50. Making fun of a resident's appearance					
51. Swearing at a resident					
52. Assisting another nursing assistant with perineal care and holding the resident down so tightly that it causes bruises					
53. Teasing a resident about his disability					
54. Yelling at a resident					
55. Mocking or ridiculing a resident's behavior					
56. Not giving a dependent resident water or fluids during your shift					
57. Not intervening when an alert resident fondles a mentally confused resident					

True/False

Mark the following statements true or false.

58. T   F   The nursing assistant is responsible for determining whether abuse has occurred.

59. T   F   A change in personality may be a sign of abuse.

60. T   F   A nursing assistant cannot be charged with abandonment as long as she notifies the nurse when she walks off the job.

61. T   F   Abuse may result from a caregiver who feels stressed, frustrated, and fatigued.

62. T   F   A nursing assistant who witnesses abuse and does not report it may be held as guilty as the abuser.

63. T   F   Follow only those facility policies with which you agree. If you think a policy is wrong, do not follow it.

64. T   F   The standard of care involves doing what a reasonable, prudent worker of similar education would do in a given situation.

65. T   F   Neglect may be accidental or deliberate.

66. T   F   Tell the residents and families when you are short of staff so they understand why you are running behind.

67. T   F   One resident hits another resident. This is an example of resident-to-resident abuse.

68. T   F   Involuntary seclusion is a form of treatment used for bad behavior.

69. T   F   The nursing assistant is responsible for protecting and respecting the rights of only those residents who are part of his assignment.

Developing Greater Insight

70. A confused resident regularly refuses his bath. It is not uncommon for the resident to put on the same dirty clothes every day. Explain why it is all right to bathe the resident and change his clothes. Explain why the resident's rights are not being violated by bathing him and changing his clothes. How can you bathe him and put clean clothes on him without agitating the resident?

_____

_____

_____

_____

_____

71. A nursing assistant does not look at a resident's care plan, and does not realize that the resident must be repositioned every two hours. The resident develops a large Stage III pressure ulcer. Was the nursing assistant negligent? Did the nursing assistant deliver care that met or exceeded the standard of care? Why or why not?

_____

_____

_____

_____

_____

72. A nursing assistant goes home sick in the middle of the shift. The nurse rearranges the assignments to ensure that all residents are cared for. At the end of the shift, you realize you have forgotten to care for Mr. Stone. You find him asleep in the chair in his room. He has been incontinent and his clothing is soiled. You do not know if he ate lunch. What action will you take?

_____

_____

_____

_____

_____

73. Rearrange the letters to form a sentence in the lower grid. (Keep the letters in the same column; skip a column for a space between words.)

	E	I	L	M		I	N	S		E	E				
	P	E	N	F		E	E	D	E	P	E	A	D	E	H	T
B	S	R	O	G	O	T	S	T	E	H	M	N	L	T	N	Y
				■												
■								■								
■				■						■	■	■	■	■	■	■

CHAPTER 6

Communication and Interpersonal Skills

KEY POINTS

- Many factors influence communication.
- Health care workers communicate with many people verbally, in writing, and through gestures, touch, and body language.
- The four elements of communication are the sender, message, receiver, and feedback.
- Using goal-oriented communication involves deciding what you want to accomplish and focusing on a topic.
- People with disabilities should be treated the way you like to be treated. Some people with disabilities have special communication needs.
- Courtesy is important when answering the telephone in the health care facility.

ACTIVITIES

Vocabulary

Define the following by selecting the correct term from the list provided here.

aphasia	expressive aphasia	prosthesis
attending behavior	feedback	receiver
barrier	global aphasia	receptive aphasia
dysarthria	message	sender
empathy	paraphrasing	sympathy

1. A method of restating the message communicated to you in clear, simple terms. _____

2. Feeling very sorry for someone because of their physical condition or situation. _____

3. The person for whom a message is intended. _____

4. An artificial body part. _____

5. A condition in which the resident has a speech disorder because the speech center in the brain has been damaged. _____

6. The information the sender wants to communicate. _____

7. A condition in which the speech center in the brain has been damaged; residents with this condition have trouble understanding what is spoken to them. The resident may also have trouble reading and understanding gestures. _____

8. The person who originates communication. _____

9. Behavior used to improve the transfer of verbal communication. _____

10. Confirmation that a message was received as it was intended by the sender. _____

11. Inability to speak or understand. _____

12. A condition that is often caused by a head injury or stroke in which the resident has weakness or paralysis of the lips, tongue, or throat. _____

13. Something that interferes with communication. _____

14. Understanding how someone else feels. _____

15. A condition in which the speech center in the brain has been damaged; residents with this condition have difficulty saying what they want to say. They may also have trouble with gestures and writing. _____

Yes or No

Do the words and the body language send the same message? Circle Y for yes and N for no.

16. Y N Sharon says she cares a great deal about her residents. She seldom makes eye contact.

17. Y N Grace shows caring by never discussing her personal life with her coworkers in front of the residents.

18. Y N Mrs. Long calls Susan into the room as she passes by. Susan asks how she can help, then bends to the resident's level, making eye contact while Mrs. Long speaks.

19. Y N Tim asks Miss Rogan about her outing with her family last weekend, then stands with his hands on his hips while she discusses her activities.

20. Y N Karen says, "Good morning!" and greets Mrs. Lim with a hug.

21. Y N Terry and Kerry say they care about the residents, then talk over them while giving care.

22. Y N Mrs. King is upset. Tina says, "I'm sorry to hear that. Tell me about it." She pulls up a chair, leans forward, and takes Mrs. King's hand.

23. Y N John enters the room and asks the resident how he is this morning. As the resident responds, John goes to the window to open the drape. He watches the children across the street for several minutes while the resident is speaking.

24. Y N Casey, Terry, and Linda say the residents are their primary concern. They discuss their dates of last weekend while they are feeding residents in the dining room.

25. Y N Jose describes himself as a caring nursing assistant. He often interrupts residents when they are speaking.

26. Y N Maria says she cares about the residents' feelings. She stands about five feet away when speaking with them, and seldom makes eye contact.

27. Y N Tony rubs the side of his head and says he has a headache.

28. Y N Mrs. Conner has turned her wheelchair toward the window, sits with her arms and legs crossed, and says she was happy to meet her new daughter-in-law.

29. Y N Chris paces back and forth, rubbing her hands together, while she says she is looking forward to transferring to another facility.

30. Y N Amy makes a face when you feed her and says she hates stew.

31. Y N Mrs. Hill has used her call signal at least four times in the past hour. Jackie rolls her eyes when she asks the resident how she can help her.

32. Y N Tony grimaces when he moves, but says he is not having pain.

33. Y N Mr. Peel says he is not in a hurry to shower and get ready for his appointment. He taps and drums his fingers on the overbed table while the nurse is speaking.

34. Y N Joan and Marcia are known as kind, compassionate nursing assistants. While making a bed, they talk excitedly about preparing a special family dinner for the upcoming holiday. They ask the resident, Mrs. Hensley, what she liked to cook for her family, and how she prepared her favorite dishes.

35. Y N Kate says she wants to make a difference in the residents' lives. She finishes her work early and goes to room 302 to help the ladies apply lotion and nail polish.

Short Answer

Write your answers in the spaces provided.

36. List at least five guidelines that you feel are important for having a conversation.

   _____
   _____
   _____
   _____
   _____

37. List five components of attending behavior.

   _____
   _____
   _____
   _____
   _____

38. List five barriers to communication.

   _____
   _____
   _____
   _____
   _____

39. List at least 10 guidelines that are important for communicating with residents who have vision loss.

   _____
   _____
   _____
   _____
   _____
   _____
   _____
   _____
   _____
   _____

40. List at least 10 guidelines that are important for communicating with residents who have hearing loss.

   _____
   _____
   _____
   _____
   _____

----

41. List at least 10 guidelines that are important for communicating with residents who have disabilities.

Completion

Complete the following statements by selecting the correct term from the list provided here.

anger	cues	identify	objects	sadness	substitutes
articulate (speak)	double	lengthy	one	see	talking
caring	hand	lightly	patronizing	slang	tone
clearly	happiness	loudness (volume)	rushed	specific	two
cover	hearing				

42. When communicating verbally, remember to

    control the _____ of your voice.

    control your voice _____.

    be aware of the way you _____.

    avoid _____ meanings.

    not use informal language or _____.

43. The pitch, inflection, and loudness of your voice can communicate a message of _____, _____, _____, or _____.

44. When communicating with a resident who is hard of hearing,

    make sure the resident can _____ you.

    stand on the resident's _____ side.

    do not _____ your mouth when speaking.

    speak _____, distinctly and naturally.

    use _____ gestures and body language to help express your meaning.

45. When communicating with a resident who is visually impaired,

    describe the environment and _____ around the resident to establish a frame of reference.

    touch the resident _____ on the hand to avoid startling him or her.

    be _____ when giving directions.

    when entering a room, _____ yourself and state your purpose.

    assist the resident to use _____ books, if desired.

46. With the disoriented resident,

    ask the resident to do only _____ task at a time.

    use word _____ if they have meaning for the resident.

    be specific, and show respect for the resident by not being _____.

    avoid appearing _____.

    avoid _____ explanations.

    offer the resident one of _____ choices.

    use nonverbal _____ freely and respectfully.

Developing Greater Insight

47. Sister Kellenhofer from St. Gregory's Church called at 11:00 a.m. on March 11 to ask how Mrs. Riley was doing. She asked to speak with the nurse, Karen Staley, RN, who was doing a treatment and could not come to the phone. Sister Kellenhofer asked that the nurse return her call. Her telephone number is 555-6237. How do you communicate this information? Complete the following form to demonstrate your understanding of this task.

```
┌──────────────────────────────────────────┐
│  To                         ☐ URGENT      │
│  Date_____Time_____  A.M.     │
│                                  P.M.     │
│        WHILE YOU WERE OUT                 │
│  From_____     │
│  Of_____     │
│  Phone_____     │
│         Area Code      Number      Ext.   │
│  ┌─────────────────┬─┐┌──────────────┬─┐  │
│  │ Telephoned      │ ││ Please call  │ │  │
│  ├─────────────────┼─┤├──────────────┼─┤  │
│  │ Came to see you │ ││ Wants to see │ │  │
│  │                 │ ││ you          │ │  │
│  ├─────────────────┼─┤├──────────────┼─┤  │
│  │ Returned your   │ ││ Will call    │ │  │
│  │ call            │ ││ again        │ │  │
│  └─────────────────┴─┘└──────────────┴─┘  │
│                                           │
│  Message _____    │
│  _____    │
│  _____    │
│  _____    │
│  _____    │
│  _____    │
│  _____    │
│  Signed _____    │
└──────────────────────────────────────────┘
```

48. **Your Message is this:**

    7% _____ **+ 38%** _____ **+ 55%** _____, _____, _____ **= Total Communication**

49. Read the following poem about body language. What parts of the body does it refer to? What does it mean? Many long-term care residents have difficulty speaking and cannot communicate with words, so they use body language. Likewise, we communicate with residents and other staff through our own expressions and body language. How does this poem apply to the long-term care resident? Can we learn anything from it?

Messengers

They express anger; That is easily detected. They express hopelessness; When we feel dejected.
They express delight; When we achieve. They express sorrow; When we grieve.
They express victory; When we win. They express forgiveness; For an imagined sin.
They express confusion; When we don't perceive. They express appreciation; For what we receive.
They express happiness; For all we hold dear. They express fright; When we encounter a fear.
They express disappointment; When we lose. They express indecision; When we must choose.
They express patience; For a child. They express excitement; When our imagination runs wild.
They express love; It's perfectly clear. They speak a language; For all to hear.
In one fluid motion; As they part. The hands become Messengers of the heart.
To really know a person; If this is your goal. Look deep into their eyes; The Messengers of the soul.*

*Courtesy of Marilyn Sossamon, LPN. Used with permission.

---

50. Mrs. Little is crying and upset. The doctor has told her that her condition will continue to deteriorate. She will not get any better. The resident's daughter said, "Don't worry about it, mother. It will be all right. I love you anyway." With that, the daughter left the facility to go home. Mrs. Little said that her daughter does not know what she is talking about. After all, the daughter does not have to live inside her body. Why is this such a poor response? What can the nursing assistant learn from it?

51. Mr. Perry's daughter asks you what her father's vital signs were this morning. She wants to know "how he is doing." How will you respond? What information can you disclose to her?

_____

_____

_____

_____

52. The resident in 512 is very sick with congestive heart failure. She has oxygen, a catheter, and is receiving IV medication. She has an advance directive and does not want heroic measures. The nurse said she may not live through the shift. The resident has many nursing needs and staff are going in and out frequently. The resident's family members are also in the facility, and the room gets crowded. The family steps out into the hallway, whispers, and cries from time to time. A visitor sees all the activity in the room and asks you what is going on. How will you respond?

_____

_____

_____

_____

53. Rearrange the letters to form a sentence in the lower grid (Keep the letters in the same columns; skip a column for a space between words.)

A	L		R	Y			D	D		T	S			
I	E		T	I	S	I	B	E	L	E	O	Y		T
H	L	I	A	Y	S	A	S	T	N	I	T	S		B
H	E	W	D	E	S	A	N	I	R	N	S	T	A	T

54. Rearrange the letters to form a sentence in the lower grid (Keep the letters in the same columns; skip a column for a space between words.)

M	O		D			A			S	O	A	
H	A	K	G	A	A	G	E	M		Y	O	U	G
L	A	R	E	U	S	U	R	E	S	B	S	D	Y	T
W	E	N	S	S	M	E	N	D	E	E	N	D	R	E

CHAPTER 7

Observations, Recording, and Reporting

KEY POINTS

- The nursing assistant communicates with other members of the health care team verbally and in writing.
- Observations about the resident are reported to the nurse for assessment and action.
- The nursing assistant records information about the resident in the medical record in writing or by using the computer.
- The nursing assistant will use the senses of sight, hearing, smell, and touch to make valuable observations.
- Signs can be seen or observed. Symptoms are things the resident tells you.
- Objective observations are factual. Subjective observations are based on what you think or what the resident tells you.
- The medical record is a factual, permanent record of the resident's progress and care.
- The medical record is a legal document and entries in it must be accurate and complete.
- Understanding medical terminology and medical abbreviations is important if you are to communicate well with other members of the health care team.

ACTIVITIES

Vocabulary

1. Complete the crossword puzzle.

Across

3 a notebook or binder containing the resident's information, observations, information about care given, and the resident's response to care

5 Health Insurance Portability and Accountability Act

7 factual observations

9 Observations that may or may not be factual; these observations are based on what you think or information the resident gives you, which may or may not be true

10 describes what is wrong with the resident

13 One part of the Health Insurance Portability and Accountability Act applies to resident _____ and confidentiality in written records and reports.

14 _____ of care means that all staff are working on the same goals, using the same approaches, 24 hours a day to benefit the residents.

Down

1 the element that provides the meaning of the word

2 things residents notice about their conditions and tell you; these things cannot be detected or confirmed by using your senses

4 a shortened form of a word

6 the word element at the beginning of a word

8 the word element ending a word

11 things that you observe by using your senses

12 The medical _____ is a legal document of resident information that can be subpoenaed and used in court.

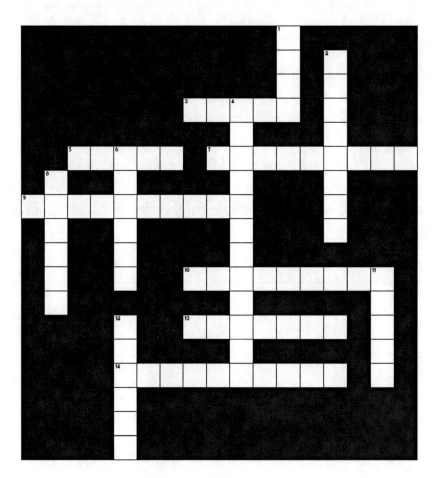

Completion

Complete the statements regarding safety practices by selecting the correct term from the list provided here.

accurate	late entry	protect
chronological	list	report
communicate	medical terminology	signature
complete	need to know	space
fax machine	not given	title
flow-sheet charting	password	unauthorized

2. If you forget to chart something, follow your facility policy for making a _____ note on the chart.

3. According to the Health Insurance Portability and Accountability Act, all health care workers must _____ the resident's records and information from access by _____ persons.

4. According to the Health Insurance Portability and Accountability Act, resident information is provided to workers on a _____ basis.

5. If you will be initialing a form, such as a flow sheet, make sure that you sign the initial key with your full _____ and _____.

6. When documenting on a computer, never give your _____ to others.

7. Make sure that documentation of your care is _____ and _____.

8. Draw a single line through unused _____ at the end of a sentence.

9. Nursing personnel will receive some type of _____ at the beginning of every shift.

10. You will _____ with others frequently throughout the shift.

11. You may use the _____ to transmit printed information from one location to another over telephone lines.

12. Entries in the chart are made in _____ order, by date and time.

13. Many facilities use _____ to document routine care.

14. Blank spaces on the medical record indicate that care was _____.

15. In the health care facility, _____ is used to describe body parts, procedures, orders, measurements, treatments, activities, time, and place.

16. Each facility will have a _____ of abbreviations approved for use in charting.

Matching

Name the sense used to determine the following information. Each sense may be used more than once.

17. _____ radial pulse

18. _____ body odor

19. _____ rash

20. _____ blood pressure

21. _____ blood in the urine

22. _____ green beans are salty

23. _____ movable lump under the skin

24. _____ wound drainage has foul odor

25. _____ skin is hot

26. _____ resident appears cyanotic

27. _____ bruises

28. _____ lemonade is sweet

29. _____ resident is coughing

30. _____ resident grimaces on movement

31. _____ red area on a bony prominence

32. _____ appetite 25% for lunch

a. seeing
b. hearing
c. smelling
d. touching
e. taste

33. _____ wheezing when the resident breathes

34. _____ dry skin

35. _____ perspiration (sweating)

36. _____ complaints from the resident

37. _____ coffee is cold and bitter

38. _____ resident is crying

39. _____ change in the way a resident walks

40. _____ smoke in hallway

a. seeing
b. hearing
c. smelling
d. touching
e. taste

Differentiation

41. Differentiate between signs and symptoms by placing an X in the appropriate column.

Observation	Sign	Symptom
nausea		
vomiting		
diarrhea		
sore throat		
incontinence		
restlessness		
dizziness		
cold, clammy skin		
elevated blood pressure		
anxiety		
cough		
pain		
fever		
abdomen distended		
constipation		
rapid pulse		

42. Differentiate subjective from objective reporting by placing an X in the appropriate column.

Observation Reported to Nurse	Subjective Reporting	Objective Reporting
Resident made a face. She probably does not like her food.		
Resident found on floor. States, "I slipped."		
Resident has a bruise on her hand and a skin tear on her elbow.		
Resident is rubbing her arm. It must hurt.		
Resident's urine has a foul odor. There are threads of mucus in the toilet.		
Resident is smiling. She is not having pain.		
Resident refused lunch. She probably was not hungry.		
Resident is sweating. Her skin is hot.		
Resident has been passing gas. She must be constipated.		
Resident has a fever and is shivering.		
Resident cannot find his room. His Alzheimer's must be worsening.		

Matching

Match each time with its equivalent on the 24-hour clock.

43. _____ 3:13 p.m.

44. _____ 12:43 a.m.

45. _____ 9:10 p.m.

46. _____ 12:22 p.m.

47. _____ 5:15 a.m.

48. _____ 10:38 a.m.

49. _____ 8:03 p.m.

50. _____ 11:25 a.m.

51. _____ 6:20 p.m.

52. _____ 9:00 a.m.

53. _____ 4:32 p.m.

54. _____ 2:30 a.m.

a. 2422   j. 1315
b. 1222   k. 2300
c. 2003   l. 0515
d. 0900   m. 1243
e. 1315   n. 1820
f. 0230   o. 1513
g. 0043   p. 1038
h. 1125   q. 2110
i. 1438   r. 1632

Completion

Complete each statement as it relates to charting by selecting the correct term from the list provided here.

abbreviations	entry	pencil
after	erase	read
blank	facts	spell
color	legibly	title

55. Use the correct _____ of ink.

56. Date and time each _____.

57. Print or write _____.

58. _____ each word correctly.

59. Do not chart in _____.

60. Do not use correction fluid or _____ information.

61. Always chart _____ giving care.

62. Leave no _____ spaces.

63. Use only facility-approved _____.

64. Chart the _____, not your opinion.

65. _____ what you have documented.

66. Sign each entry with your first initial, last name, and _____.

True/False

Mark the following statements true or false.

67. T   F   Report subjective observations to the nurse promptly.

68. T   F   Changes that seem insignificant may indicate a problem.

69. T   F   Symptoms are things you identify with your senses.

70. T   F   Chart care that you know is supposed to be given, such as turning every two hours, even if you did not have time to do it.

71. T   F   Use short, concise phrases in your charting.

72. T   F   If you forget to chart something, make a late entry in the record.

73. T   F   Begin setting your priorities when you listen to report at the beginning of the shift.

74. T   F   It is all right to read residents' charts to satisfy your curiosity.

75. T   F   The HIPAA regulations protect all individually identifiable health information in any form.

76. T   F   Computers used for documentation have audit trails that track the machine name, user, date, time, and exactly which medical records were accessed based on the user identification.

77. T   F   Documentation of information about resident elimination is not important.

78. T   F   Observation of the resident is a continuous process.

79. T   F   A common maxim in health care is, "If it is not charted, it was not done."

80. T   F   Long-term care facilities seldom use computers for documentation.

Completion

Define the following abbreviations in the spaces provided.

81. stat _____

82. BID _____

83. PRN _____

84. UTI _____

85. PO _____

86. QID _____

87. c̄ _____

88. HS _____

89. c/o _____

90. NPO _____

91. w/c _____

92. TPR _____

93. OOB _____

94. B/P _____

95. HOB _____

96. ✓ _____

97. @ _____

98. ↑ _____

99. O_2 _____

100. AM _____

Developing Greater Insight

Answer questions 101–104 based upon the following situation.

Lynette has been running behind all day. Mr. Stepanik had an emergency in the morning, which caused her to get behind, and she could not get caught up. All her assigned residents were bathed and fed. At the end of the shift, she completes her documentation and checks the flow sheets, which are complete. She documents intake and output, baths, and meal intake on her assigned residents. She charts that she toileted Mrs. Sturm every two hours because she knows this is the care she was supposed to provide. In fact, she did not take Mrs. Sturm to the bathroom at all. The resident was not incontinent, so she reasoned that this omission was harmless. She did not inform the nurse that the resident had not voided at all during her shift. After completing her documentation, she left for the day. Six hours after she left the facility, Mrs. Sturm was crying and complaining of abdominal pain. She was found to have a very distended abdomen. The nurse emptied her bladder with a catheter and obtained more than a quart of bloody, foul-smelling urine.

101. Was Lynette's documentation accurate and complete? _____

102. Could Lynette have managed things differently when she realized she could not get her work done? If so, how?

_____

_____

_____

_____

103. Did her actions harm Mrs. Sturm? Explain your answer.

_____

_____

_____

_____

104. Are there legal implications of this situation?

_____

_____

_____

_____

CHAPTER 8

Body Mechanics, Moving and Positioning Residents

KEY POINTS

- Good body mechanics are used when lifting and moving residents and other heavy objects.
- Ergonomics is a method of fitting the job to the worker to prevent injuries.
- Residents must always be positioned in good body alignment.
- The primary cause of pressure sores is lack of oxygen and circulation to the skin, caused by pressure.
- Pressure ulcers are easier to prevent than to treat.
- Wearing a back support belt does not make you stronger; avoid lifting more weight than you would if you were not wearing the belt.
- Pressure ulcers are declines; most pressure ulcers are preventable.
- Residents with current pressure ulcers or a history of healed pressure ulcers are at high risk for additional skin breakdown.
- Documentation of turning and positioning residents is very important; accurate documentation verifies that care was given as ordered, and according to the plan of care.
- Lying in the fetal position for a prolonged period of time greatly increases the risk of complications.
- Positioning residents in the semiprone and semisupine positions relieves pressure from all major bony prominences.

ACTIVITIES

Vocabulary

1. Complete the puzzle by finding the words listed.

4 letters	6 letters	8 letters	10 letters	13 letters
DRAW	CRADLE	PRESSURE	ERGONOMICS	INSTANTANEOUS
FOOT	SUPINE		SEMISUPINE	
	TRAUMA	9 letters		15 letters
5 letters		ABRASIONS	11 letters	CONTRAINDICATED
FETAL	7 letters	DECUBITUS	PROMINENCES	
PRONE	FOWLERS	MECHANICS		
	LATERAL	SEMIPRONE		

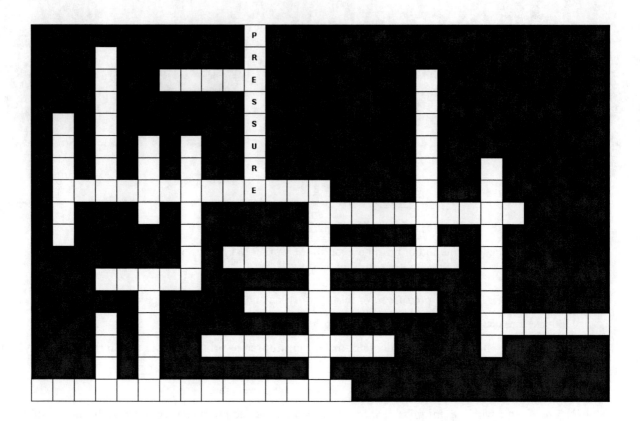

Logical Order

Place the beginning procedure actions in the proper order. Number each action 1 through 15.

2. _____ Apply gloves if contact with blood, moist body fluids (except sweat), secretions, excretions, or non-intact skin is likely.

3. _____ Assemble equipment and take it to the resident's room.

4. _____ Explain what you are going to do and how the resident can assist. Answer questions about the procedure.

5. _____ Set up the necessary equipment at the bedside. Open trays and packages. Position items within easy reach. Avoid positioning a container for soiled items in a manner that requires crossing over clean items to access it.

6. _____ Apply a gown, mask, and eye protection if splashing of blood or moist body fluids is likely.

7. _____ Ask visitors to leave the room and advise them where they may wait.

8. _____ Provide privacy by closing the door, privacy curtain, and window curtains.

9. _____ Wash your hands or use an alcohol-based hand cleaner.

10. _____ Knock on the resident's door and identify yourself by name and title.

11. _____ Lower the side rail on the side where you are working.

12. _____ Position the resident for the procedure. Ask an assistant to help, if necessary, or support the resident with pillows and props. Make sure the resident is comfortable and can maintain the position throughout the procedure. Drape the resident for modesty, even if you and the resident are alone in the room.

13. _____ Raise the bed to a comfortable working height.

14. _____ Identify the resident by checking the identification bracelet or other method according to facility policy.

15. _____ Apply a gown if your uniform will have substantial contact with linen or other articles contaminated with blood, moist body fluid (except sweat), secretions, or excretions.

Place the procedure completion actions in the proper order. Number each action 16 through 28.

16. _____ Open the privacy and window curtains.

17. _____ Inform visitors that they may return to the room.

18. _____ Elevate the side rails, if used, before leaving the bedside.

19. _____ Check to make sure the resident is comfortable, and in good alignment.

20. _____ Report completion of the procedure and any abnormalities or other observations.

21. _____ Replace the bed covers, then remove any drapes used.

22. _____ Document the procedure and your observations.

23. _____ Remove other personal protective equipment, if worn, and discard according to facility policy.

24. _____ Return the bed to the lowest horizontal position.

25. _____ Leave the resident in a safe and comfortable position, with the call signal and needed personal items within reach.

26. _____ Wash your hands or use an alcohol-based hand cleaner.

27. _____ Wash your hands or use an alcohol-based hand cleaner.

28. _____ Remove gloves.

True/False

Mark the following statements true or false.

29. T F Wearing the back support belt makes you stronger.

30. T F Pressure ulcers are easier to prevent than they are to treat.

31. T F Pressure increases blood flow and nourishment to the skin.

32. T F Heel and elbow protectors do not relieve pressure.

33. T F Most pressure ulcers are preventable.

34. T F If you must turn or change direction, twist at the waist.

35. T F When positioning the resident in the Fowler's position, the head of the bed is elevated 45 degrees.

36. T F Pressure ulcers are declines.

37. T F Your strongest muscles are in your legs and arms.

38. T F The presence of a risk factor makes deterioration inevitable.

39. T F Tucking the top linen in tightly promotes foot drop.

40. T F Ergonomics is a method of fitting the worker to the job.

41. T F Having a current pressure ulcer or a history of healed pressure ulcers means the resident is at high risk for further pressure ulcer development.

42. T F Stage II pressure ulcers are areas in which the skin is lost and the subcutaneous fat and muscle are exposed.

43. T F Shearing is rubbing the skin against another surface, such as bed linen.

44. T F The skin is the largest organ of the body.

45. T F Blisters and abrasions that occur as a result of moving residents are Stage II pressure ulcers.

46. T F Cumulative trauma disorders occur from repeated stress and strain over a period of months to years.

47. T F Turn dependent residents at least every four hours.

48. T F The pressure from wrinkles and crumbs in bed linen can cause skin breakdown.

49. T F Elevating the head of the bed increases the risk of skin breakdown.

50. T F Friction involves moving the skin in one direction while the underlying bones move in the opposite direction.

51. T F Check residents' skin daily and report abnormalities to the nurse promptly.

52. T F Using plenty of soap, powder, and cornstarch helps maintain residents' skin integrity.

53. T F Hair and nails are part of the skin system.

54. T F Pressure ulcers are not painful.

55. T F Bedfast residents should remain in bed with side rails up and the bed in the highest horizontal position at all times.

56. T F Pad bony areas, such as between the knees and ankles to keep skin surfaces from rubbing together.

57. T F A Stage I ulcer is a red area that does not go away after the pressure has been removed for 30 minutes.

58. T F Nutrition and hydration have no effect on pressure ulcer risk.

59. T F Skin that is supple and well hydrated will not break as easily as dry skin.

60. T F Pillows are useful for resident positioning.

Short Answer

Briefly explain the reasoning behind each of the following statements.

61. The nursing assistant should use leg and shoulder muscles instead of back muscles for moving residents and heavy objects. Why?

_____

_____

_____

_____

62. Nursing assistants must be conscientious about resident positioning. Why?

_____

_____

_____

_____

63. The semisupine and semiprone positions are different from the lateral position. Why is using these positions advantageous to residents?

_____

_____

_____

_____

64. You should remain in the room for a period of time when the resident first uses the prone or semiprone position. Why is this important?

_____

_____

_____

_____

65. Residents must be positioned in one of the Fowler's positions during and after meals and tube feedings. Why is this necessary?

_____

_____

_____

_____

66. Residents with low risk of pressure ulcers may develop pressure ulcers quickly if they become ill and bedfast. Why?

_____

_____

_____

_____

67. Moving resident(s) with a lift sheet is better for the resident(s) and the nursing assistant(s). Why?

_____

_____

_____

_____

68. Documentation of turning and positioning residents is very important. Why?

_____

_____

_____

_____

69. Residents should be positioned in good body alignment. Why?

_____

_____

_____

_____

70. Lying in the fetal position for a prolonged period of time greatly increases the risk of complications. Why?

_____

_____

_____

_____

Identification

71. In the space provided on the left, name the position pictured on the right.

a. _____

b. _____

c. _____

72. Identify at least six pressure areas in this picture.

a. _____

b. _____

c. _____

d. _____

e. _____

f. _____

73. Identify at least six pressure areas in this picture.

a. _____

b. _____

c. _____

d. _____

e. _____

f. _____

74. Identify at least six pressure areas in this picture.

   a. _____

   b. _____

   c. _____

   d. _____

   e. _____

   f. _____

75. Identify at least six pressure areas in this picture.

   a. _____

   b. _____

   c. _____

   d. _____

   e. _____

   f. _____

76. a. State what this figure represents. _____

   b. What is the most common way that this problem occurs?_____

   c. What problem does it cause for the resident? _____

   d. How can it be prevented? _____

Developing Greater Insight

Answer the following questions based on this situation.

Mr. Howard is an alert, dependent resident who is quite obese. He was admitted with a Stage III pressure ulcer that took a long time to heal. He often gets red, angry-looking spots under his arms, and under the loose skin on his chest and abdomen. When this occurs, the nurses treat the areas with an antifungal cream. The care plan states that his skin must be dried well after bathing, and notes that the resident must be turned by two or more assistants every two hours or more often using a lift sheet. The resident sometimes repositions himself after staff turn him. On one such occasion, he developed a Stage I pressure ulcer. He is to be encouraged to lean forward or push up to relieve pressure when he is sitting in a wheelchair. The resident's skin is loose and rubs together in many areas of his body. The care plan states that all staff should encourage fluids. The resident does not like water, and usually refuses it even though his water pitcher is filled several times a shift.

77. Is Mr. Howard at high risk of developing pressure ulcers? Why or why not?

_____

_____

_____

_____

78. Why is it important to dry the resident's skin folds well after bathing?

_____

_____

_____

_____

79. What is the benefit of using a lift sheet to move the resident?

_____

_____

_____

_____

80. What can be done to maintain the resident's position?

_____

_____

_____

_____

81. The resident does not like water. What can the nursing assistant do to maintain good fluid intake for this resident?

_____

_____

_____

_____

82. Rearrange the letters to form a sentence in the lower grid. (Keep the letters in the same columns; skip a column for a space between words.)

	A		V		E				A		A	
P	R	E	A	E	E	R	E	T	H	R	N	E	O	S
P	Y	E	E	R	N	A	S	O	U	T	C	E	R	H
E	R	R	S	S	U	T	T	I	E	L	R	T	T	T

CHAPTER 9

Assisting Residents with Mobility

KEY POINTS

- A transfer belt should always be used when moving residents, unless contraindicated.
- A transfer involves moving a resident from one location to another.
- Sitting on the side of the bed is called dangling; this is the first step in the transfer procedure if the resident has been bedfast.
- Lock the brakes on the bed and wheelchair before transferring the resident.
- Move the footrests out of the way if the resident is transferring into a wheelchair.
- A key to maintaining stability of the wheelchair is positioning the large part of the front caster wheels facing forward.
- Always lock the brakes during transfers into and out of a wheelchair, and when the chair is parked.
- Position the resident in the wheelchair in good body alignment.
- The resident's legs must be supported on the footrests or the floor when the resident is seated in a wheelchair.
- The mechanical lift is a two-person device.
- A resident with good upper body strength can use a sliding board to transfer from the bed to a wheelchair and back.
- The wheelchair must fit the resident properly for comfort, safety, and to reduce the use of restraints.
- Pressure ulcers can develop when a resident is seated in the wheelchair; pressure relief must be provided.
- The wheelchair is a mobility device, not a transportation device. The resident should propel the chair independently whenever possible.
- The care plan will list purposeful activities for maintaining residents' ambulation ability.
- Residents may need canes, walkers, or crutches for balance, stability, and support during ambulation.

ACTIVITIES

Vocabulary

Find the words in the accompanying puzzle. In phrases, only the words in italics are hidden in the puzzle. Define each word or phrase.

a	g	q	t	r	a	n	s	f	e	r	f	a	g
c	t	a	u	b	d	o	d	j	a	k	m	a	p
o	d	a	s	a	e	w	a	m	k	b	i	g	a
l	a	a	x	t	d	f	h	q	u	t	m	w	c
o	n	o	e	i	r	j	x	l	j	t	u	n	e
s	g	z	i	s	c	o	a	j	a	q	y	o	m
t	l	o	q	m	o	t	s	j	o	e	a	i	a
o	i	i	m	v	i	g	a	t	h	z	f	s	k
m	n	w	v	o	n	n	i	t	o	h	p	i	e
y	g	z	n	i	z	e	m	a	r	m	x	c	r
z	e	u	d	n	g	l	q	b	t	o	y	n	h
k	e	i	t	z	x	b	h	c	l	m	p	i	q
t	l	a	n	e	u	r	y	s	m	p	z	h	b
s	c	h	a	i	r	f	a	s	t	f	c	h	y

1. ambulation _____

2. aneurysm _____

3. *ataxic* gait _____

4. atrophy _____

5. chairfast _____

6. colostomy _____

7. dangling _____

8. gait _____

9. gastrostomy _____

10. incision _____

11. pacemaker _____

12. *quad* cane _____

13. transfer _____

14. *sliding* technique _____

Corrections

Correct the statements that are wrong by drawing a line through the incorrect word or words. Write the corrections under them as needed. Do not make any changes to correct statements.

15. Know the resident's capabilities before attempting a transfer.

_____

16. Instruct residents to lock their hands behind your neck during the transfer.

_____

17. Use a lift sheet for standing transfers.

_____

18. It is not necessary to explain the transfer to confused residents.

_____

19. Transfer residents toward the weakest side.

_____

20. A transfer belt is not routinely used in the long-term care facility.

_____

21. Residents with IVs, drainage bags, and feeding tubes are transferred by nurses.

_____

22. Give the resident only the assistance he needs to transfer.

_____

23. Before transferring the resident, position the bed in the highest horizontal position.

_____

24. Always use correct body mechanics when transferring the resident.

_____

25. Position the wheelchair at a 90-degree angle, with the small part of the front wheels facing forward.

_____

26. Stand close to the resident during the transfer.

_____

27. Make sure the resident is wearing footwear appropriate to the surface of the floor.

_____

28. A gait belt must always be used to transfer residents with newly implanted medication pumps.

_____

29. The wheelchair must have removable armrests when the sliding board is used.

_____

30. Reclining chairs help improve the residents' orientation to the environment.

_____

31. Residents cannot develop pressure ulcers when sitting in a chair.

   _____

32. For safety, the wheelchair must be used correctly, and fit the resident.

   _____

33. The wheelchair is strictly a transportation device.

   _____

34. When transporting a resident by stretcher, the safety belt need not be fastened if the side rails are up.

   _____

35. For best results, ambulation should be goal-oriented.

   _____

36. Residents with an ataxic gait need a narrow base of support.

   _____

37. When ambulating residents, hold the gait belt with an overhand grasp.

   _____

38. The quad cane is the least stable type of cane.

   _____

True/False

Mark the following statements true or false.

39. T F   A transfer belt should be used to transfer residents with no ability to bear weight.
40. T F   The buckle of the transfer belt should be fastened in the front.
41. T F   The transfer belt is applied under the resident's clothing.
42. T F   The transfer belt is contraindicated for a resident with an abdominal aneurysm.
43. T F   The transfer belt may be removed after the transfer is complete.
44. T F   Wheelchairs are manufactured so that one size fits all.
45. T F   There should be one fingerwidth between the resident's knees and the wheelchair seat.
46. T F   The resident's legs may dangle in the air, but should not drag the floor when in the wheelchair.
47. T F   Some residents need restraints because they are in wheelchairs that do not fit.
48. T F   Staff should always push residents' wheelchairs.
49. T F   When pushing a wheelchair, enter the elevator facing forward, then turn around and back out.
50. T F   When assisting with ambulation, stand directly behind the resident.
51. T F   The resident's cane and the weak leg move forward at the same time.
52. T F   Crutches provide a sturdy base of support.
53. T F   The front legs of the walker should strike the floor first.
54. T F   The mechanical lift may be safely used by one nursing assistant.
55. T F   If the resident will be using a sliding board, dress him in blue jeans.

Identification

56. Look carefully at each picture. List the corrections that should be made in each.

Corrections: a. _____
             b. _____
             c. _____
             d. _____

Corrections: e. _____
             f. _____
             g. _____
             h. _____

Corrections: i. _____
             j. _____
             k. _____
             l. _____

Corrections: m. _____

n. _____

o. _____

p. _____

Completion

Complete the following statements in the spaces provided.

57. Before beginning a transfer, determine if additional _____ is needed.

58. Before attempting to transfer a resident, you should learn his or her _____-bearing ability.

59. When assisting a resident to transfer into a wheelchair, make sure the footrests are _____.

60. The sling for the mechanical lift should be positioned between the resident's _____ and _____.

61. A resident who is _____ is unable to move.

62. To _____ means to turn the entire body to one side.

63. A transfer belt is also called a _____ belt.

64. When assisting with transfers, move _____ with the resident.

65. You should be able to slip _____ or _____ fingers under a properly applied gait belt.

66. Place a folded _____ in the seat of the chair if the resident is wearing a hospital gown.

67. The resident's _____ are positioned at a 90-degree angle, at the back of the wheelchair.

68. Use of the transfer belt is _____ for both the nursing assistant and the resident.

69. The resident _____ into the walker with the weak leg, then the strong leg.

Developing Greater Insight

Answer the following questions based on this situation.

You are assigned to care for Mr. Holzauer for the first time today. The resident is very tall and underweight. This confused resident can respond verbally, but his statements are not always appropriate. He responds correctly to simple commands. The care plan says he is full weight bearing, and to use a one-person transfer from bed to wheelchair. The care plan also notes that he is at high risk for skin breakdown. He has a red area on his toe. You put his socks and shoes on and he complains of pain in the toe, and asks you to remove the shoes.

70. Is it safe to transfer this resident by yourself? Why or why not?

_____

71. If you are unsure of the resident's ability to transfer, what should you do?

_____

72. Will you use a transfer belt for this transfer?

   _____

73. Since the resident is at risk of skin breakdown, are any special precautions or equipment necessary for transferring to the wheelchair?

   _____

74. Should you transfer the resident without his shoes because of the pain in his toe?

   _____

75. Is any action necessary related to the red area and pain in the toe?

   _____

76. In light of the shoe problem and pain in the toe, should you transfer this resident alone?

   _____

77. You have transferred the resident to the wheelchair with the nurse's help. When you position Mr. Holzauer's arms on the armrests, you note that his shoulders are elevated to just below his ears, and his knees are elevated higher than his thighs. What is the most likely cause of the problem?

   _____

78. Rearrange the letters to form a sentence in the lower grid.

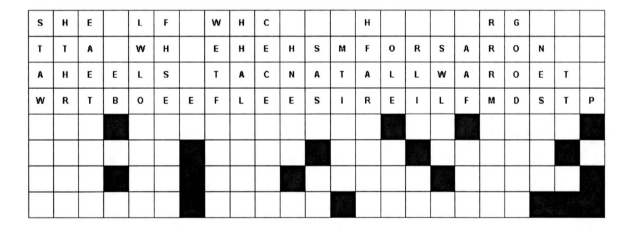

CHAPTER 10

Care of the Environment

KEY POINTS

- The resident's unit is an area for personal use.
- Respect the residents' rights when giving care and handling personal belongings.
- *Think safety* when you enter and leave the room.
- Follow your facility infection control policies for separation of clean and soiled items.
- Follow your facility policies for handling soiled linen.
- Practice the principles of standard precautions when making the bed if contact with blood, body fluids (except sweat), secretions, or excretions is likely.
- Personal protective equipment is removed after soiled linen is disposed of. The hands are washed before handling clean linen and touching other environmental surfaces.
- The nursing assistant is responsible for keeping resident rooms tidy. You may also be responsible for routine cleaning assignments that must be completed during or at the end of the shift.

ACTIVITIES

Vocabulary

Each line has four different spellings of a word or phrase from this unit. Circle the correctly spelled word.

1. blanckit	blanket	blankit	blanckat
2. bedsid stande	bed said stand	bedside stand	bedsyde stan
3. gatch handles	gash handles	gach handls	gatch hendles
4. lowebed	low bed	lobid	lower bed
5. myter	maeter	mitre	miter
6. occupyed bedmacking	occupeid bedmaking	ockupied bedmakeing	occupied bedmaking
7. hoverbed table	overbed table	ovverbed table	ovyrbed taible
8. toe pleat	toe pleet	tow pleate	toe plate
9. bathe	baeth	baith	beathe
10. linnen hamper	linnin hamper	linen hammper	linen hamper
11. nurishment list	nourishment list	nurrishmant list	nourichment list
12. medication room	madication room	medicashun room	medication roome
13. utelety room	utility room	youtility room	utylity room
14. pantrie	pantrey	panttry	pantry
15. unockupyed bed	unoccupied bed	unocupied bed	unocupyd bed
16. labratory specimin	laboratory specimen	labratry spesimen	labertorie spessiman
17. kleening assignment	cleening assinement	cleaning assignment	kleaning assinement

Matching

Match the terms and description.

18. _____ hospital bed
19. _____ mat
20. _____ soiled utility
21. _____ shower room
22. _____ nurses' station
23. _____ dining room
24. _____ linen cart
25. _____ clean utility
26. _____ pantry

a. used to take clean linen into hallways
b. placed on the floor for some residents who are at risk of rolling out of bed
c. food storage
d. used for storage of new, clean, or sterile supplies
e. used for cleaning soiled supplies
f. used for resident meals
g. most important piece of furniture in the resident's room
h. used for resident bathing
i. work area for nursing personnel; medical records stored here

Identification

Locate and identify each of the areas in the floor plan (below). Write the name of the area on the line below. Then, state one fact or precaution for each area that is *not noted* in questions 18 through 26.

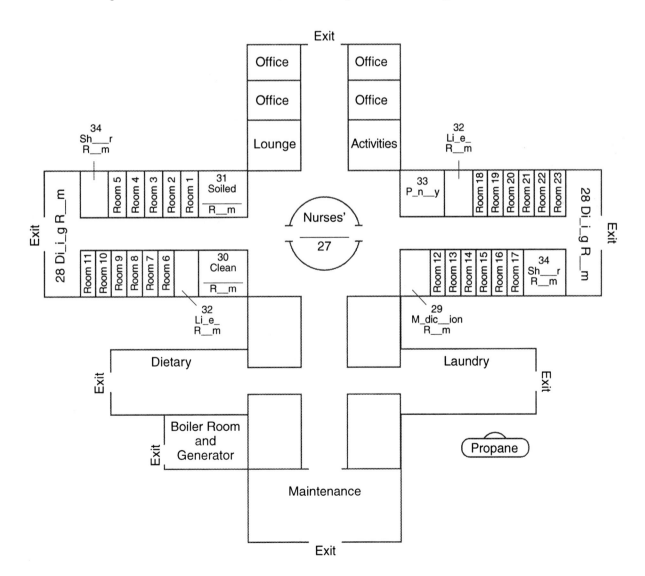

27. nurses' _ _ _ _ _ _ _

_____

_____

28. di _ i _ g r _ _ m

_____

_____

29. m _ dic _ _ ion r _ _ m

_____

_____

30. clean _ _ _ r _ _ m

_____

_____

31. soiled _ _ _ _ _ _ _ r _ _ m

_____

_____

32. li _ e _ r _ _ m

_____

_____

33. p _ n _ _ y

_____

_____

34. sh _ _ _ r r _ _ m

_____

_____

Completion

Complete the table in the spaces provided.

Method of Bedmaking	Procedure Variations	Rationale
35. _____	a. _____	c. Easier and faster for the nursing assistant.
	b. Used for making all types of beds.	d. More comfortable for the resident.
36. Occupied bed	a. _____	b. _____
		c. _____
37. Closed bed	a. _____	d. _____
	b. Pillow may be covered or placed on top of spread, depending on facility policy.	e. _____

c. Open end of the pillowcase faces
away from the door.

---

38. _____   a. _____

    b. _____

c. Procedure is used when the
resident is temporarily out of bed.

d. Resident or nursing assistant can
easily and quickly cover the
resident upon return to bed.

True/False

Mark the following statements true or false.

39. T F Before making a bed, lower it to the lowest horizontal height.

40. T F Apply gloves before removing wet linen; remove gloves when finished making the bed.

41. T F A fitted sheet may be used on the mattress in place of a flat sheet.

42. T F Position the lift sheet so it goes between the resident's waist and knees.

43. T F Before making the unoccupied bed, arrange the linen in the order of use.

44. T F Clean linen for making the bed should be placed on the bedside stand.

45. T F Place soiled linen on the overbed table or floor.

46. T F When making an occupied bed, roll the bottom linen until it is against the resident's back, then turn
the resident.

47. T F Shake linen as you remove it from the bed.

48. T F Leave the soiled linen hamper outside the door with the lid open.

49. T F Always check the bed linen for lost items, such as dentures, glasses, and hearing aids.

50. T F The top linen should be loosened slightly at the foot when the bed is occupied.

51. T F Raise the side rails when you are finished making the bed so the resident cannot go back to bed.

52. T F Use the gatch handle on the left to raise the head of the bed.

53. T F The overbed table is a soiled area.

54. T F Bend at the waist to make a low bed.

55. T F Check the call signal daily.

56. T F The call signal should be within the resident's reach at all times, except if the resident is confused.

57. T F If the resident's body is exposed, he or she is covered with a bath blanket, even if the door and
curtains are closed.

58. T F When making the occupied bed, raise the side rails if you must step away from the bedside.

Identification

Identify the following.

59. Personal care items in residents' rooms must be labeled with each resident's name. Identify items that must be labeled with an "L" (label). Identify items that do not require a label with an "N" (no label).

   a. toothbrush _____

   b. dresser _____

   c. bedspread _____

   d. water pitcher _____

   e. wastebasket _____

   f. bedside chair _____

   g. urinal _____

   h. overbed table _____

   i. bedpan _____

   j. wash basin _____

   k. bedside stand _____

   l. emesis basin _____

   m. drinking glass _____

   n. straw _____

   o. clean washcloth _____

   p. clean towel _____

   q. hair brush _____

   r. pillow _____

   s. comb _____

60. Identify what is wrong with each picture. State what to do to correct it.

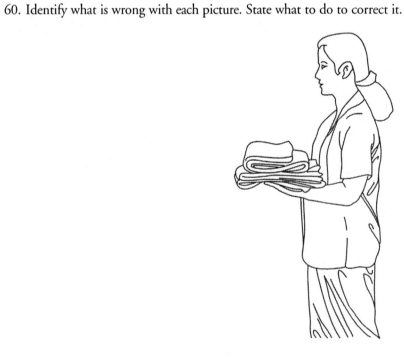

   a. error _____

   b. correction _____

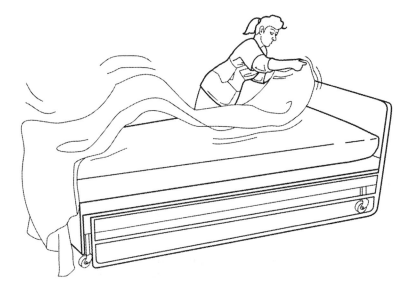

c. error _____

d. correction _____

61. What is wrong with the figure on the left? Correct it in the figure on the right by writing the names of the articles in the correct location.

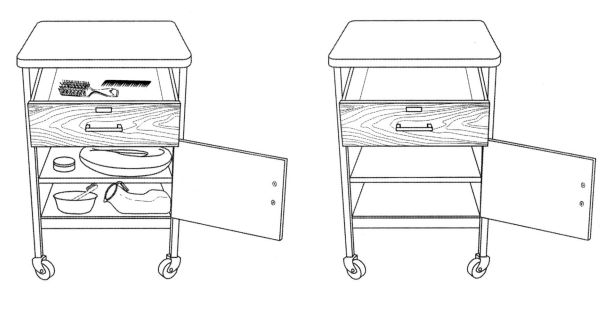

a. error _____

b. correction _____

Developing Greater Insight

Answer the following questions based on this situation.

You must make 12 complete beds today as part of your assignment. If a bed becomes soiled, you must change it a second time. Based on this assignment, answer the following questions.

62. Why should one side of the bed be made completely before moving to the other side?

_____

_____

63. How should the pillow be placed on the bed? Why?

_____

_____

64. Mrs. Gianossi has been ill and is weak. She gets up in a chair for an hour, then returns to bed to rest. After changing the sheets, you will probably have to straighten the bed several more times on your shift. You have decided to make an open bed for this resident. Why?

_____

_____

65. Mr. Hofmaier is a dependent resident who transfers with the mechanical lift and two assistants. He goes down for a nap from 2:00 to 4:30 p.m., then gets up for supper. He soils the bed at 2:45 p.m., immediately before your shift ends. Will you change the bed or leave it for the next shift? If you elect to change the bed, what type of bedmaking procedure will you use? Why?

_____

_____

66. A resident has been discharged, and you must make a closed bed. How will you position the overbed table after making the bed?

_____

_____

67. You accidentally brought an extra sheet into Miss Geary's room. Your facility policy does not permit you to leave extra linen in residents' rooms. Should you use it when you make the bed in the room next door? Put it back on the linen cart? If not, what will you do with the sheet?

_____

_____

68. Your facility keeps a box of gloves in a wall dispenser in each room. A bedfast resident has been incontinent, and you must make an occupied bed. You bring all your supplies to the room and stack them in the order of use. You raise both side rails and elevate the bed to the highest horizontal position. The top linen is not wet, so you cover the resident with a bath blanket and fold the top linen down. Then you lower the side rail on one side to begin. You remember you must apply gloves for handling the wet linen and discover that the box of gloves is empty. Should you proceed without gloves? If not, what action will you take?

_____

_____

69. Rearrange the letters to form a sentence in the lower grid. (Keep the letters in the same columns; skip a column for a space between words.)

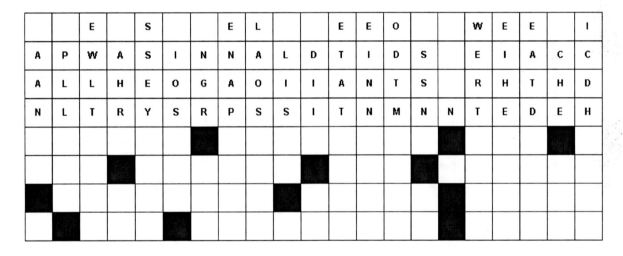

70. Rearrange the letters to form a sentence in the lower grid. (Keep the letters in the same columns; skip a column for a space between words.)

CHAPTER 11

Personal Care Skills

KEY POINTS

- Good personal hygiene is essential to proper health.
- Activities of daily living are things people do every day to meet their health and hygienic needs.
- The nursing assistant assists residents to meet health and hygienic needs when they are unable to take care of these needs independently.
- Oral hygiene is the cleaning of the resident's mouth, teeth, gums, and tongue.
- Special oral hygiene is given frequently to residents who are unconscious, NPO, tube feeders, or receiving oxygen.
- Dentures are artificial teeth that require special care and handling.
- Bathing is done to cleanse the skin, stimulate circulation, provide exercise, and refresh and relax the resident.
- Bath time is an excellent time to make observations of the resident's skin and body.
- Bath water temperature is checked with a thermometer. A comfortable temperature for bathing is 105°F.
- When bathing residents, wash from clean to dirty areas.
- The bed bath is given to residents who are on complete bedrest; it involves cleaning the resident's entire body.
- The partial bath involves washing the resident's face, hands, underarms, back, and genital area.
- When giving perineal care to a female, wash from front to back. Avoid rubbing back and forth.
- When giving perineal care to a male, wash from the tip of the penis to the rectum.
- Massaging the resident's back is comforting, refreshing, and stimulating to circulation. Giving a back rub helps prevent skin breakdown.
- In most agencies, the nursing assistant does not cut fingernails or toenails.
- Antiembolism hose increase blood flow to the legs and prevent blood clots, edema, and other complications.
- A prosthesis is used to replace a missing body part.
- The resident's self-esteem is enhanced when she is dressed and well groomed.

ACTIVITIES

Vocabulary

Unscramble the words and define them.

1. Scare H _____

2. dbe thab _____

3. runtesed _____

4. tninntineoc _____

5. hanithb talsweres _____

6. isnab eesism _____

7. lqueap _____

8. xalail _____

9. artipal hatb _____

10. MceraA _____

11. cxcoyc _____

12. ripe-acer _____

13. abht omelcpet _____

14. naitmiemlobs tocsgknis _____

15. psutm csko _____

16. notefaron reca _____

17. igalten erae _____

18. eyeghin _____

19. gimnnro earc _____

20. sitivaceit vinlig fo yiadl _____

Word Search

Read the following definitions, then find and circle each word in the puzzle.

i	n	j	f	s	i	s	e	m	e	n	t
o	n	e	s	w	o	a	y	d	i	k	o
u	p	c	h	f	j	b	d	s	p	s	o
g	a	c	o	y	o	s	a	r	g	c	t
e	w	y	l	n	y	b	o	v	n	e	h
n	i	f	z	t	t	s	o	z	y	u	b
e	h	a	c	r	t	i	h	z	c	q	r
i	w	l	d	h	u	d	n	j	z	a	u
g	k	n	e	u	u	b	y	e	b	l	s
y	v	s	d	n	z	g	a	h	n	p	h
h	i	i	i	s	g	r	d	d	o	c	t
s	r	x	s	e	r	u	t	n	e	d	e

21. false teeth

22. decay-causing substance

23. basin used for oral care procedures

24. artificial body part

25. personal cleanliness

26. inability to control elimination

27. instrument for brushing teeth

28. used to hold water for bathing procedures in bed

Completion

Complete the following statements in the spaces provided.

29. Before giving a back rub, _____ the lotion in _____.

30. The temperature of bath water should be _____ °F.

31. Dentures should be handled _____ to prevent damage.

32. The denture cup should be labeled with _____.

33. When brushing a resident's teeth, hold the brush at a _____-degree angle against the teeth.

34. Brush all _____ of the teeth.

35. When brushing dentures, line the sink with _____.

36. You need not _____ the residents' skin with a towel when waterless bathing products are used.

37. A partial bath involves cleansing of the hands, face, _____, buttocks, and _____.

38. Do not use _____ near the eyes.

39. When cleaning the eyes, wipe from the _____ to _____.

40. Wash the female resident's perineum from _____ to _____.

41. Apply lotion to the residents' feet to care for dry skin, but never apply lotion _____.

42. When washing the hair, give the resident a _____ to protect the eyes.

43. When giving perineal care to a female resident, _____ the washcloth so you use a _____ section for each stroke.

44. The water temperature in the whirlpool tub is usually set at _____ °F to _____ °F.

45. Always cover the resident with a _____ during bathing procedures.

46. Never leave the resident _____ in the tub or shower.

47. Always fasten the _____ when the resident uses the whirlpool lift chair.

48. Avoid using hair products designed for _____ on African American residents.

49. Persons of color need extra _____ on the hair at all times. This product should be applied to the _____ and not the hair.

50. Applying _____ immediately after bathing seals moisture in the skin, preventing dryness.

51. Apply the principles of _____ when assisting with personal care procedures.

52. When bathing a resident in the tub or shower, turn the cold water _____ first and _____.

True/False

Mark the following statements true or false.

53. T   F   Keeping the mouth clean reduces the incidence of pneumonia.

54. T   F   Residents need mouth care weekly if they have no teeth and no dentures.

55. T   F   Rinse the residents' dentures well under hot water.

56. T   F   Heat the bag bath package for approximately four to five minutes before bathing the resident.

57. T   F   Keep the resident's body completely covered during transport to and from the shower room.

58. T   F   The jets in the whirlpool tub may harbor dangerous pathogens, and must be disinfected well.

59. T   F   Discard the bag bath washcloths by flushing them down the toilet.

60. T   F   When giving perineal care to a resident who has a urinary catheter, wash the perineum, then use the washcloth to scrub back and forth on the catheter to cleanse it well.

61. T F Bag bath should not be used on residents with dry skin.

62. T F If you will be using liquid soap from a dispenser mounted on the wall to bathe the resident, dispense the soap directly into the bath water.

63. T F Pour liquid soap directly into the whirlpool tub to wash the resident.

64. T F The whirlpool activity provides a cleansing action.

65. T F Oil the scalp of African American residents, then brush the oil down into the hair.

66. T F Do not apply antiembolism hosiery over open areas, fractures, or deformities.

67. T F Antiembolism hosiery should be worn at all times.

68. T F Keeping the residents' skin moisturized and well lubricated helps reduce the risk of injury.

69. T F When giving a back rub, massage red areas well.

70. T F Discard disposable razors in the trash can.

71. T F Wear gloves when shaving residents with a disposable razor.

72. T F If you accidentally cut a resident with the razor, apply pressure with an alcohol sponge.

73. T F The skin on the feet of elderly persons heals slowly if injured.

74. T F Use an orange stick for cleaning residents' fingernails.

75. T F Elevate the residents' legs for at least 20 minutes before applying antiembolism hosiery.

Developing Greater Insight

76. Mrs. Alopaeus has severe contractures. You cannot spread her legs to wash her genital area. What are the potential consequences of forcing the legs apart? How will you give peri-care to this resident?

_____

_____

77. Mr. Baumeister has diabetes. His toenails are long, jagged, and dirty. He asks you to cut them. He says they cause pain when he wears shoes. Your facility requires residents to wear shoes when out of bed. What action will you take? Will you put shoes on the resident?

_____

_____

78. Rearrange the letters to form a sentence in the lower grid. (Keep the letters in the same columns; skip a column for a space between words.)

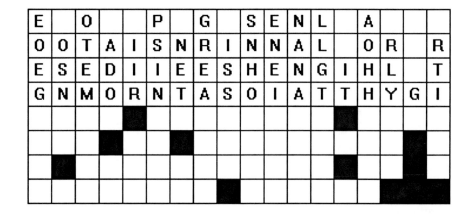

CHAPTER 12

Comfort, Pain, Rest, and Sleep

KEY POINTS

- All humans need comfort, rest, and sleep for physical and emotional well-being, health, and wellness.

- Comfort is a state of physical and emotional well-being.

- Pain is a state of discomfort that is unpleasant for the resident; it is always a warning that something is wrong.

- Residents' responses to pain may be related to culture.

- Body language may be the first (and only) clue that a resident is having pain.

- Relieving pain is an important nursing responsibility.

- The resident's self-report of pain is the most accurate indicator of the existence and intensity of pain, and should be respected and believed.

- Residents may have pain when they are laughing, talking, or sleeping; vital signs may be normal.

- Pain rating scales are important tools for communication. They prevent subjective opinions, provide consistency, eliminate some barriers to pain management, and give the resident a means of describing the pain accurately.

- The incidence of drug addiction is very low in individuals with persistent pain who take narcotic analgesics.

- Rest is a state of mental and physical comfort, calmness, and relaxation. The basic needs of hunger, thirst, elimination, and pain must be met before effective rest is possible.

- Sleep is a period of continuous or intermittent unconsciousness in which physical movements are decreased and the mind and body rest.

- Sleep is a basic need. Adequate sleep is necessary for the body and mind to function properly.

- Less sleep is required as people age.

- Rapid eye movement sleep restores mental function.

- Spirituality and religion can provide great comfort and support during times of illness and emotional distress.

- Spirituality and religion are not the same thing.

- Spirituality includes our perceptions of our place in the universe, belief in a higher power (if any), ideas about our responsibilities to others, and our fears and beliefs about living and dying.

- Caring for residents during very private moments is a privilege. The nursing assistant should show sensitivity when residents express spiritual concerns.

ACTIVITIES

Vocabulary

1. Complete the crossword puzzle.

Across

3 _____ pain is usually the result of tissue damage.

5 pain that develops as a result of an amputation

6 pain that moves from one location to another

8 pain-relieving medication

12 a state of discomfort that is unpleasant for the resident

13 pain lasting for more than six months

Down

1 nonrapid eye movement sleep

2 Sleep _____ occurs when the resident does not get enough sleep.

4 Residents may describe the intensity of pain by using a pain rating _____.

7 rapid eye movement sleep

9 a state of physical and emotional well-being

10 a period of continuous or intermittent unconsciousness in which physical movements are decreased

11 a state of mental and physical comfort, calmness, and relaxation

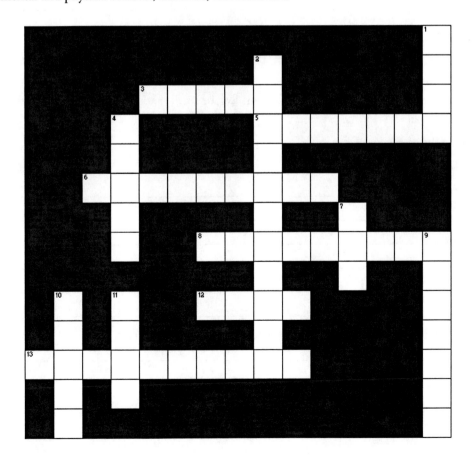

Completion

Complete the sentences to show that you understand each type of pain listed.

Type of Pain	Description
2. Acute pain	Occurs _____. It usually results from _____. Typically, acute pain decreases over time, as _____.
3. Persistent pain	Persistent pain lasts _____. An older term for this type of pain is _____.
4. Phantom pain	Phantom pain occurs as a result of _____. The pain is _____ imaginary.
5. Radiating pain	Radiating pain moves from _____.

Short Answer

Briefly complete the following.

6. List eight factors that may interfere with the resident's ability to sleep.

    a. _____

    b. _____

    c. _____

    d. _____

    e. _____

    f. _____

    g. _____

    h. _____

7. List eight observations that you see, hear, feel, or smell that should be reported to the nurse regarding a resident's pain.

    a. _____

    b. _____

    c. _____

    d. _____

    e. _____

    f. _____

    g. _____

    h. _____

8. How is the resident's outward expression of pain affected by culture?

    _____

9. List at least eight controllable or uncontrollable factors that affect the resident's comfort, rest, and sleep.

    a _____

    b. _____

c. _____

d. _____

e. _____

f. _____

g. _____

h. _____

10. What is the purpose of the pain rating scale?

_____

11. Why is using the pain rating scale a key to accurate pain evaluation?

_____

12. Why is uninterrupted REM sleep important?

_____

13. List 10 things the nursing assistant can do to enhance the residents' comfort, rest, and sleep, and relieve pain.

a. _____

b. _____

c. _____

d. _____

e. _____

f. _____

g. _____

h. _____

i. _____

j. _____

True/False

Mark the following statements true or false.

14. T   F   The nurse's assessment is always more accurate than a resident's self-report of pain intensity.

15. T   F   A resident must be lying in bed to rest properly.

16. T   F   Comfort is a state of well-being.

17. T   F   Full-color dreams occur during the NREM phase of the sleep cycle.

18. T   F   Elderly adults require about five to seven hours' sleep per day.

19. T   F   Phantom pain is psychological pain.

20. T   F   The body repairs itself during sleep.

21. T   F   A resident who is resting may pray or say the rosary.

22. T   F   If a resident is sick, hunger and thirst do not interfere with the ability to rest.

23. T   F   Lack of privacy may affect the resident's comfort and ability to rest.

24. T   F   There are two phases of the NREM sleep cycle.

25. T   F   The resident passes into REM sleep within approximately 60 to 90 minutes after falling asleep.

26. T   F   Spirituality can provide comfort and support to residents during times of illness and emotional distress.

27. T F The nursing assistant should help the residents identify, define, and analyze spiritual truths.

28. T F Spirituality and religion are the same thing.

29. T F Body language is often the first clue that a resident is having pain.

30. T F A confused resident may be able to clearly describe his pain.

31. T F Pain management is the nurses' responsibility.

32. T F Residents with severe pain often become addicted to the pain medications.

33. T F Relieving discomfort helps reduce pain and anxiety.

34. T F Adult residents may need frequent rest periods during the day.

35. T F Getting enough sleep and rest enables residents to function at their highest level.

36. T F The body's metabolic needs increase during sleep.

37. T F Residents who do not get enough REM sleep may be more tired during the day.

38. T F The nursing assistant must be prepared to assist residents with solving personal problems, such as financial worries.

39. T F Some residents may appear comfortable while having severe pain.

40. T F Pain is a major preventable public health problem.

41. T F Pain does not affect quality of life.

Developing Greater Insight

Use your critical thinking skills to identify at least one benefit to the resident of the listed nursing assistant actions pertaining to comfort, pain, rest, and sleep.

Nursing Assistant Action	Benefit to Resident
42. Ensuring privacy, reducing noise, eliminating unpleasant odors, and adjusting the temperature, lighting, and ventilation are major nursing assistant responsibilities.	
43. Handling the resident gently, assisting the resident to assume a comfortable position, using pillows and props for repositioning, giving a back rub, and providing emotional support are routine tasks that are very important when a resident is having pain.	
44. Meeting the resident's needs for basic needs of hunger, thirst, elimination, pain, and good hygiene.	
45. Scheduling care to prevent awakening the resident during sleep, keeping the environment comfortable, and reducing noise.	

46. Mrs. Tinsley just returned to the facility following hip replacement surgery. The resident uses the FACES pain scale (Figure 12-1). The nurse gave her pain medication at 3:15 p.m. At 4:30, you answer the call signal. The resident is crying, points to the frowning face ("Hurts whole lot"), and tells you her pain is number four. You look at the resident's hip area, but do not see anything visibly wrong, then hand her the box of tissues. What does this pain level suggest? What action will you take first? What actions can you take to assist this resident?

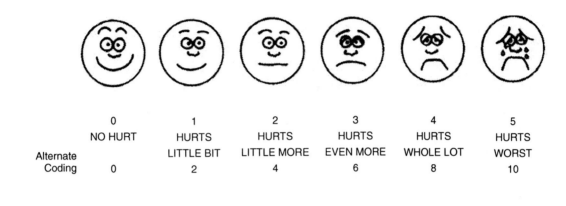

	0 NO HURT	1 HURTS LITTLE BIT	2 HURTS LITTLE MORE	3 HURTS EVEN MORE	4 HURTS WHOLE LOT	5 HURTS WORST
Alternate Coding	0	2	4	6	8	10

_____

_____

_____

Answer the following questions based on this situation.

Your resident, Mrs. Vasquez, has spinal stenosis and frequently complains of pain. The nurse alternates an injection for pain with an oral medication every two hours.

47. Mrs. Vasquez is laughing and visiting with her family. When you enter the room with fresh ice water, she tells you she is in pain. Can a resident who is laughing and visiting be having pain? Explain your answer.

_____

48. Mrs. Vasquez refuses her supper tray. She tells you she is having too much pain to eat. What action should you take?

_____

49. Mrs. Vasquez tells you she feels better now, and would like to eat. The kitchen has closed for the evening. What action should you take?

_____

50. Why do you think that hunger, thirst, pain, and need to use the bathroom affect the residents' comfort and ability to rest or sleep?

_____

51. Mrs. Vasquez cannot sleep. She tells you that her low back really hurts. What nursing assistant measures can you take to make her more comfortable?

_____

CHAPTER 13

Nutrition and Hydration

KEY POINTS

- Water, vitamins, minerals, carbohydrates, fats, and proteins are essential for good health.
- The USDA food pyramid recommends a specific number of servings from each of the six food groups each day.
- Five common categories of diets are served in health care facilities.
- Therapeutic diets are planned by the licensed dietitian to meet a resident's specific medical needs.
- The nursing assistant is responsible for preparing residents for meals, serving trays, feeding residents, and removing trays after residents have eaten.
- Tube feeding, intravenous feeding, and hyperalimentation are alternative methods of feeding residents who have special needs.
- Dysphagia is a condition in which the resident has difficulty swallowing and is at risk for choking. Special techniques are used to prevent aspiration of food and fluids.
- Residents in long-term care facilities can and do develop malnutrition and dehydration. The nursing assistant must be aware of at-risk residents and take steps to prevent these conditions.
- Measuring fluid intake and output is an important responsibility of the nursing assistant.
- The nurse is responsible for recording intake for tube feedings and medications. The nursing assistant is responsible for recording all other fluid intake, including fluids residents consume in the dining room and at activities.
- The nursing assistant applies principles of medical asepsis when passing fresh drinking water to residents.

ACTIVITIES

Vocabulary

Fill in the following definitions by selecting the correct term from the list provided here.

calorie-controlled	low-fat	pureed
clear liquid	mechanical soft	regular
diabetic	mechanically altered	sodium-restricted
full liquid	no concentrated sweets	soft or bland
low cholesterol		

1. The _____ diet restricts the total number of calories served to the resident; it is usually served to overweight residents.

2. The texture of a _____ diet is changed to meet the needs of residents with chewing, swallowing, or digestive problems.

3. A _____ diet has been prepared with no sodium or limited sodium.

4. A _____ diet is low in fat for residents who have heart, blood vessel, liver, and gallbladder disease.

5. A _____ diet has been blenderized to a smooth consistency.

6. The _____ diet is a normal diet based on the food groups in the food pyramid.

7. A _____ diet is high in water and carbohydrates, with little nutritive value.

8. A _____ diet contains foods that are low in residue, with limited or no seasoning.

9. A _____ diet is a regular diet that is not calorie restricted, but free sugar, fruit in sugary syrup, and most regular desserts are not served.

10. The _____ diet includes clear and milk-based liquids and is served to residents who have digestive disorders.

11. A _____ diet provides reduced fat and cholesterol to residents who have heart, blood vessel, liver, and gallbladder disease.

12. A _____ diet has been calculated by the dietitian to meet the needs of a resident who has diabetes mellitus; the diet limits free sugar and some other foods.

13. The _____ diet is finely ground or chopped for residents who have chewing or swallowing problems.

Matching

Match the terms and description.

14. _____ inorganic compounds in food used to build body tissues

15. _____ elasticity of skin

16. _____ administering sterile liquid and nutrients into a vein with a needle

17. _____ abnormal drowsiness or sleepiness

18. _____ food products such as butter and oil that are used for heat and energy production

19. _____ limiting the total amount of fluid the resident can have in a 24-hour period

20. _____ diagram that provides a guide to eating a well-balanced diet

21. _____ an order to encourage the resident to drink as much liquid as possible

22. _____ metric unit of measure used in health care facilities; 30 cc equals one ounce

23. _____ chemical substances in food that are necessary for life

24. _____ an estimated measurement of all the liquid the resident takes in and all the fluid he or she loses in a 24-hour period

25. _____ a tube inserted into the nose and threaded through the esophagus into the stomach; used for feeding or medical procedures

26. _____ foods that produce heat and energy in the body

27. _____ organic substances in food that are necessary for normal body function

28. _____ inadequate nutrition due to poor diet, or inability to absorb nutrients

a. cubic centimeter
b. food pyramid
c. vitamins
d. fats
e. nasogastric tube
f. intake and output
g. supplemental feedings
h. malnutrition
i. force fluids
j. proteins
k. minerals
l. nutrients
m. dysphagia
n. lethargy
o. carbohydrates
p. strict I&O
q. intravenous feedings
r. dehydration
s. fluid restrictions
t. milliliter
u. turgor
v. gastrostomy

29. _____ surgical procedure in which a feeding tube is placed directly into the resident's stomach, with the end extending through the abdominal skin

30. _____ serious condition resulting from inadequate water in the body

31. _____ nutrient in food that builds and repairs tissues

32. _____ an accurate measurement of all the liquid the resident takes in and all the fluid lost in a 24-hour period

33. _____ a metric unit of measure used in health care facilities; 30 mL equals one ounce; the equivalent of one cubic centimeter

34. _____ nourishments given to the resident in addition to meals to meet special nutritional needs

35. _____ difficulty swallowing food and liquids

Completion

Complete the chart by filling in the number of servings in each food group.

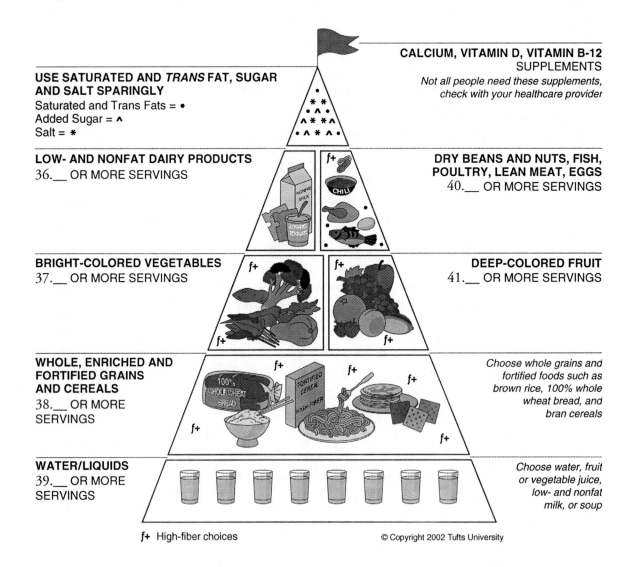

CALCIUM, VITAMIN D, VITAMIN B-12
SUPPLEMENTS
Not all people need these supplements, check with your healthcare provider

USE SATURATED AND *TRANS* FAT, SUGAR AND SALT SPARINGLY
Saturated and Trans Fats = •
Added Sugar = ∧
Salt = *

LOW- AND NONFAT DAIRY PRODUCTS
36.__ OR MORE SERVINGS

DRY BEANS AND NUTS, FISH, POULTRY, LEAN MEAT, EGGS
40.__ OR MORE SERVINGS

BRIGHT-COLORED VEGETABLES
37.__ OR MORE SERVINGS

DEEP-COLORED FRUIT
41.__ OR MORE SERVINGS

WHOLE, ENRICHED AND FORTIFIED GRAINS AND CEREALS
38.__ OR MORE SERVINGS

Choose whole grains and fortified foods such as brown rice, 100% whole wheat bread, and bran cereals

WATER/LIQUIDS
39.__ OR MORE SERVINGS

Choose water, fruit or vegetable juice, low- and nonfat milk, or soup

f+ High-fiber choices   © Copyright 2002 Tufts University

Complete the following statements in the spaces provided.

42. If you serve nourishments to a resident who is on I&O, you must

_____.

43. A mechanically altered diet may be served to residents who have problems with _____ or

_____.

44. When a resident has orders for a calorie count, all food intake is accurately _____ at each meal.

45. Residents with _____ have difficulty swallowing food and fluids and are at high risk of aspiration.

46. Sodium-restricted diets are some of the most _____ diets to follow.

47. Unless otherwise ordered, most residents should consume _____ mL to _____ mL of fluid each day.

48. There are _____ major food groups in the USDA Food Guide Pyramid.

49. When serving a meal tray to a visually impaired or blind resident, describe the location of food items compared with a _____.

50. Keep food _____ during transportation to maintain temperature and prevent contamination.

51. Serve all _____ before returning used trays to the food cart.

52. Food must be served promptly to maintain _____.

53. Unless otherwise instructed, position all residents in the _____ position for meals and for 30 to 60 minutes after meals.

54. Residents who are at greatest risk of _____ may forget what they ate, or if they ate, or forget to eat altogether.

55. To increase food intake and prevent weight loss, create a _____ dining atmosphere for the residents.

56. Check food temperature by _____.

57. When a resident is being fed by tube, elevate the head of the bed at least _____ to _____ degrees while the feeding is running and for 30 to 60 minutes thereafter.

58. _____ is a very serious condition in the elderly. Residents who are at high risk for this condition have not consumed enough liquid to support their minimum body functions.

59. One ounce of liquid is the approximate equivalent of _____ mL.

60. One quart of liquid is the approximate equivalent of _____ mL.

61. When recording I&O, count all fluids and food items that become _____ at room temperature.

Calculation

Document the following on the I&O worksheet, then calculate the total fluid intake in mL for each resident.

62. Mrs. Holiday drank 3 ounces water + 4 ounces coffee + 3 ounces juice + 240 mL milk.

Mother Teresa Care Center
Fluid Intake and Output Worksheet

Resident Name: _____   **Room:** _____

| Date | Time | Method of Adm | Intake | | | Output | | | |
			Solution	Amount	Time	Urine Amount	Other Output (specify)	Amount	Time

63. Mr. Gomez consumed 8 ounces fruit drink + 6 ounces soup + 5 ounces tea + ½ cup ice cream.

			Intake			Output			
Date	Time	Method of Adm	Solution	Amount	Time	Urine Amount	Other Output (specify)	Amount	Time

Mother Teresa Care Center
Fluid Intake and Output Worksheet

Resident Name: _____   **Room:** _____

64. Miss Stockburger consumed 300 mL water + 8 ounces supplement + 16 ounces soda + ½ cup gelatin.

Mother Teresa Care Center Fluid Intake and Output Worksheet
Resident Name: _____   Room: _____

Date	Time	Method of Adm	Intake			Output			
			Solution	Amount	Time	Urine Amount	Other Output (specify)	Amount	Time

65. Mrs. Schoebel drank 4 ounces tea + 8 ounces milk + 1 ounce cream + 4 ounces juice.

Mother Teresa Care Center
Fluid Intake and Output Worksheet

Resident Name: _____   **Room:** _____

Date	Time	Method of Adm	Intake			Output			
			Solution	Amount	Time	Urine Amount	Other Output (specify)	Amount	Time

66. Mrs. Sedala consumed a 4-ounce cup of sherbet + 12 ounces milk + 6 ounces coffee.

Mother Teresa Care Center
Fluid Intake and Output Worksheet

Resident Name: _____ **Room:** _____

			Intake			Output			
Date	Time	Method of Adm	Solution	Amount	Time	Urine Amount	Other Output (specify)	Amount	Time

67. Mr. Frahler drank a 210 mL milkshake + 10 ounces water + 5 ounces broth + 6 ounces punch.

<table>
<tr><td colspan="12" align="center">**Mother Teresa Care Center**
Fluid Intake and Output Worksheet

Resident Name: _____ **Room:** _____</td></tr>
</table>

| | | | Intake | | | Output | | | |
Date	Time	Method of Adm	Solution	Amount	Time	Urine Amount	Other Output (specify)	Amount	Time

Calculate meal intake for the residents using the following chart. Round the results to the nearest whole number.

	Food Item	Percentage of Meal
Breakfast	eggs	35%
	eggs and bacon	40%
	eggs and sausage	45%
	toast *or* cereal	30%
	milk	20%
	fruit juice	15%
Dinner and Supper	meat group, including eggs, main dish, legumes (peas, beans, soybeans)	50%
	fruit group, including dessert items	15%
	bread or cereal group	10%
	vegetable group	15%
	fluids	10%

68. For breakfast, Mr. Farago ate all the eggs and bacon, one of two pieces of toast, no milk, and all the juice. His total meal consumption is _____ %.

69. For breakfast, Miss Bazeley ate all the scrambled eggs, all the cereal with half the milk, and half the juice. Her total meal consumption is _____ %.

70. For lunch, Mrs. Heuer ate half the meatloaf, all the spinach, and half the fruited gelatin. She left all the other items on her tray. Her total meal consumption is _____ %.

71. For lunch, Mr. Calzaretta ate all the bread and all the fruited gelatin. He left all the other food items. His total meal consumption is _____ %.

72. For supper, Dr. Dill ate all the fish, all the potatoes, all the vegetable, all the bread, and all the dessert, and drank all the milk. His total meal consumption is _____ %.

73. For supper, Mrs. Ardelean ate one-quarter of the fish, half of the potatoes, and three-fourths of the vegetables, and drank all the milk. Her total meal consumption is _____ %.

Next, calculate meal intake for the same residents using the following chart. Document the intake for each resident. Compare the intake to the percentages listed for questions 68 to 73.

Calculating Percentage Consumed

Write down number of points for items eaten. If resident does not eat all food, calculate as follows:

Breakfast: toast, 2 points; eggs, 3 points
Lunch & Dinner: meat, 2 points; vegetable, 2 points; starch, 2 points

Add total points for food items eaten.
Put a zero at the end of the number for the percentage consumed.

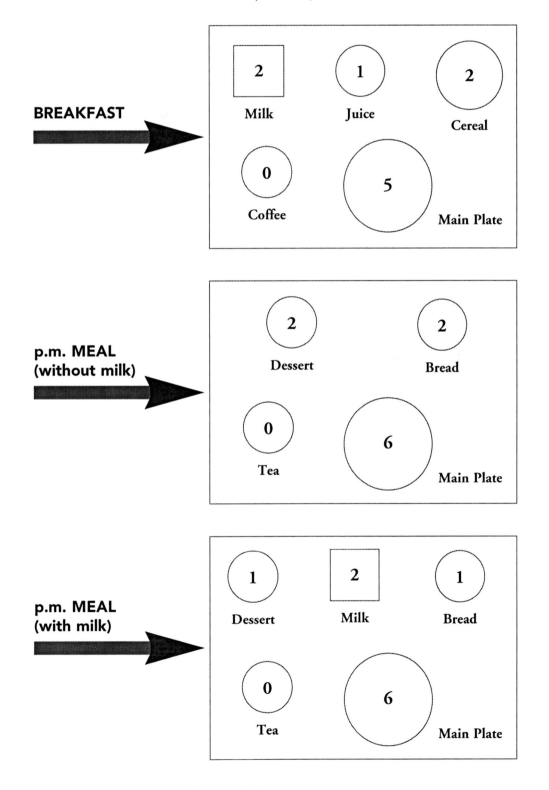

74. For breakfast, Mr. Farago ate all the eggs and bacon, one of two pieces of toast, no milk, and all the juice. His total meal consumption is _____ %.

75. For breakfast, Miss Bazeley ate all the scrambled eggs, all the cereal with half the milk, and half the juice. Her total meal consumption is _____ %.

76. For lunch, Mrs. Heuer ate half the meatloaf, all the spinach, and half the fruited gelatin. She left all the other items on her tray. Her total meal consumption is _____ %.

77. For lunch, Mr. Calzaretta ate all the bread and all the fruited gelatin. He left all the other food items. His total meal consumption is _____ %.

78. For supper, Dr. Dill ate all the fish, all the potatoes, all the vegetable, all the bread, and all the dessert, and drank all the milk. His total meal consumption is _____ %.

79. For supper, Mrs. Ardelean ate one-quarter of the fish, half of the potatoes, and three-quarters of the vegetables, and drank all the milk. Her total meal consumption is _____ %.

80. After documenting meal intake using two different methods, which do you prefer? Are they equally accurate? Is one more accurate than the other? Which is easiest to use? Why or why not?

----

81. Mrs. Espinosa is on a calorie count. You are responsible for documenting her food intake for breakfast and lunch. Calculate her meal intake using the method listed in the figure on page 95 Complete the calorie count sheet using the method listed in the figure on page 97.

Breakfast — ½ of total scrambled eggs and sausage, ½ of milk, all cereal, all juice, all coffee

The resident's total intake is _____.

Lunch — ½ hamburger patty on bun with sweet pickles and catsup, ½ spinach, ½ french fries, all ice cream, ½ tea

The resident's total intake is _____.

Diet _____

CALORIE/PROTEIN SUMMARY

RESIDENT _____ ROOM # _____

DAY 1	% 0–25	% 25–50	% 50–75	% 75–100	DAY 2	% 0–25	% 25–50	% 50–75	% 75–100	DAY 3	% 0–25	% 25–50	% 50–75	% 75–100
DATE ___/___/___					DATE ___/___/___					DATE ___/___/___				
Breakfast					**Breakfast**					**Breakfast**				
Meat					Meat					Meat				
Milk					Milk					Milk				
Fruit					Fruit					Fruit				
Starch					Starch					Starch				
Fat					Fat					Fat				
Other					Other					Other				
AM Supp.					AM Supp.					AM Supp.				
Noon Meal					**Noon Meal**					**Noon Meal**				
Meat					Meat					Meat				
Milk					Milk					Milk				
Juice					Juice					Juice				
Starch					Starch					Starch				
Vegetable					Vegetable					Vegetable				
Bread					Bread					Bread				
Fat					Fat					Fat				
Dessert					Dessert					Dessert				
Other					Other					Other				
PM Supp.					PM Supp.					PM Supp.				
Evening Meal					**Evening Meal**					**Evening Meal**				
Meat					Meat					Meat				
Milk					Milk					Milk				
Juice					Juice					Juice				
Starch					Starch					Starch				
Vegetable					Vegetable					Vegetable				
Bread					Bread					Bread				
Fat					Fat					Fat				
Dessert					Dessert					Dessert				
Other					Other					Other				
PM Supp.					PM Supp.					PM Supp.				
Total Kcal					**Total Kcal**					**Total Kcal**				
Total Pro					**Total Pro**					**Total Pro**				
Avg. for 3 days Kcal:					**Avg. Protein for 3 days:**									

PLEASE RETURN COMPLETED FORM TO NUTRITION CARE MANAGER

Developing Greater Insight

82. Mrs. Gillaspie is a very picky eater. She began losing weight, so the physician ordered weekly weights and oral nutritional supplements. These were given at 10 a.m., 4 p.m., and 9 p.m. You notice that the resident likes the supplements, but they are sweet and filling, and if the resident drinks the supplement, she does not eat her meals. You know the resident likes sweet beverages better than water, but will drink water if it is very cold with a lot of ice. You also notice that she often eats a little of the food on her meal tray, then brings other food items back to her room to eat later. Unfortunately, she often forgets to eat them, and you have had to throw things away because they were not refrigerated. The resident will eat in between meals if she likes the food. She particularly likes fruit. She dislikes meats that are difficult to chew, and dark green vegetables such as spinach and broccoli. She will eat breads if prepared with jelly or honey, but will not eat buttered bread, biscuits, or rolls.

Mrs. Gillaspie was hospitalized in January. She was diagnosed with malnutrition and dehydration. The hospital dietitian noted that she was underweight, with laboratory values suggesting malnutrition. The physician discussed the need for a gastrostomy feeding tube with the resident and family. They decided to delay the procedure and to return the resident to the long-term care facility and try to work on her weight.

When Mrs. Gillaspie returns to the long-term care facility, the dietitian is in the building for a consultant visit. The nurse informs you that they will be having a care plan meeting at 2:00 p.m. to address the resident's nutritional needs. She asks you to attend the meeting because you know the resident so well. What information will you share and/or suggest to help the team develop a care plan for this resident?

CHAPTER 14

Elimination

KEY POINTS

- The urinary system regulates water in the body and filters waste products from the blood and eliminates them from the body.

- The average adult eliminates 1,500 mL of urine from the body each day. Additional fluid is lost in respiration, perspiration, and bowel elimination.

- The nursing assistant must be professional, sensitive, and understanding when assisting residents with elimination needs.

- Incontinence is a medical problem.

- Urinary tract infections are more common in women than in men because the female urethra is shorter.

- Residents with catheters are at high risk of infection because the catheter provides an opening directly into the bladder.

- Maintaining sterility of the catheter by using aseptic technique is a very important responsibility.

- A graduate is used to accurately measure urinary output.

- Feces are a solid waste product eliminated through the digestive system.

- Constipation, fecal impaction, and diarrhea are common problems that the nursing assistant will assist with.

- The resident's self-esteem is affected by problems with elimination, and the nursing assistant must be professional, sensitive, and compassionate in meeting the resident's needs.

- An enema is an injection of fluid into the rectum to cleanse the lower bowel.

- An ostomy is a surgically created opening into the body. Several different types of ostomies are used to treat disorders of bowel elimination.

ACTIVITIES

Vocabulary

Find the words in the puzzle. In phrases, only the words in italics are hidden in the puzzle. Define each word or phrase.

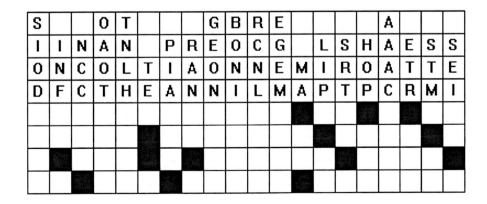

1. abdominal *distention* _____

2. anus _____

3. *aseptic* technique _____

4. bedpan _____

5. bladder _____

6. *bowel* movement _____

7. catheter _____

8. colostomy _____

9. *condom* catheter _____

10. constipation _____

11. defecation _____

12. diarrhea _____

13. *drainage* bag _____

14. enema _____

15. feces _____

16. flank _____

17. flatus _____

18. foreskin _____

19. *functional* incontinence _____

20. graduate _____

21. impaction _____

22. *indwelling* catheter _____

23. *intermittent* catheter _____

24. kidneys _____

25. *labia* majora _____

26. laboratory *requisition* _____

27. *midstream* (clean-catch) specimen _____

28. ostomy _____

29. *overflow* incontinence _____

30. penis _____

31. peristalsis _____

32. prostate _____

33. *reflex* incontinence _____

34. *retention* enema _____

35. septic _____

36. *Sims'* position _____

37. sterile _____

38. stoma _____

39. stool _____

40. *stress* incontinence _____

41. *suprapubic* catheter _____

42. ureters_____

43. urethra _____

44. *urge* incontinence _____

45. urinal _____

46. urination_____

47. voiding _____

Identification

48. Identify the equipment pictured.

    a. _____

    b. _____

    c. _____

    d. _____

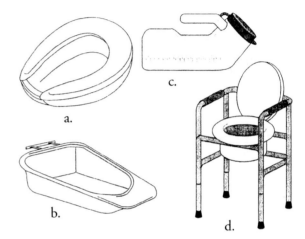

True/False

Mark the following statements true or false.

49. T F Place the used bedpan on the overbed table.

50. T F Covering the bedpan is not necessary if the bathroom is in the resident's room.

51. T F The resident's buttocks should rest on the narrow end of the bedpan.

52. T F Make sure the signal cord is within reach when a resident is using the bedpan.

53. T F Male residents use the urinal for both urinary and bowel elimination.

54. T F A dusting of powder will keep the bedpan from sticking.

55. T F Residents should be covered when using the bedpan.

56. T F You cannot position a resident on a bedpan if he is unable to lift the hips.

57. T F The urinary output may be recorded by checking the markings on the side of the catheter drainage bag.

58. T F Avoid disconnecting the closed urinary drainage system.

59. T F A resident with functional incontinence does not have the physical ability to get to the bathroom without assistance.

60. T F Loss of bowel and bladder control is a normal consequence of aging.

61. T F Apply the principles of contact precautions when assisting with elimination procedures.

62. T F Residents will have less difficulty with elimination if they are sitting (or standing) upright.

63. T F A condom catheter is an indwelling catheter.

64. T F A condom catheter should be changed daily.

65. T F Voiding frequently in small amounts is a sign of infection.

Calculation and Documentation

Document the following on the I&O worksheet, then calculate the total fluid output in mL for each resident.

66. Mr. Lieberman was incontinent one time on your shift. He voided three times in the urinal as follows: 8:00 a.m.—incontinent; 10:30 a.m.—voided 215 mL; 1:00 p.m.—voided 190 mL; 2:50 p.m.—voided 285 mL.

<table>
<tr><td colspan="10" align="center">**Mother Teresa Care Center**
Fluid Intake and Output Worksheet

Resident Name: _____ **Room:** _____</td></tr>
<tr><td rowspan="3"></td><td rowspan="3"></td><td rowspan="3"></td><td colspan="3" align="center">Intake</td><td colspan="4" align="center">Output</td></tr>
<tr><td rowspan="2"></td><td rowspan="2"></td><td rowspan="2"></td><td rowspan="2">Urine Amount</td><td rowspan="2">Other Output (specify)</td><td rowspan="2"></td><td rowspan="2"></td></tr>
<tr></tr>
<tr><td>Date</td><td>Time</td><td>Method of Adm</td><td>Solution</td><td>Amount</td><td>Time</td><td></td><td></td><td>Amount</td><td>Time</td></tr>
<tr><td></td><td></td><td></td><td></td><td></td><td></td><td></td><td></td><td></td><td></td></tr>
</table>

67. Miss Romcevich voided three times as follows: 7:15 a.m.—325 mL; 10:10 a.m.—390 mL; 1:50 p.m.—285 mL.

Mother Teresa Care Center
Fluid Intake and Output Worksheet

Resident Name: _____ Room: _____

Date	Time	Method of Adm	Intake			Output			
			Solution	Amount	Time	Urine Amount	Other Output (specify)	Amount	Time

68. Mrs. Lewis voided five times as follows: 7:40 a.m.—220 mL; 9:15 a.m.—190 mL; 11:50 a.m.—260 mL; 1:10 p.m.—205 mL; 2:30 p.m.—170 mL.

Mother Teresa Care Center
Fluid Intake and Output Worksheet

Resident Name: _____   Room: _____

Date	Time	Method of Adm	Intake			Output			
			Solution	Amount	Time	Urine Amount	Other Output (specify)	Amount	Time

69. Mr. Bugee vomited 250 mL at 7:55 a.m. He voided twice as follows: 340 mL at 10:00 a.m.; 280 mL at 1:45 p.m.

Mother Teresa Care Center
Fluid Intake and Output Worksheet

Resident Name: _____ Room: _____

			Intake			Output			
Date	Time	Method of Adm	Solution	Amount	Time	Urine Amount	Other Output (specify)	Amount	Time

70. Mrs. Hernandez had a large, involuntary, liquid stool in bed at 7:10 a.m. She voided 170 mL at 8:05 a.m.;
    240 mL at 10:40 a.m.; 200 mL at 12:05 p.m.; 265 mL at 2:35 p.m.

Mother Teresa Care Center
Fluid Intake and Output Worksheet

Resident Name: _____ Room: _____

| Date | Time | Method of Adm | Intake | | | Output | | | |
			Solution	Amount	Time	Urine Amount	Other Output (specify)	Amount	Time

71. Mr. Lim voided 310 mL at 7:15 a.m.; he was incontinent of a moderate amount at 10:00 a.m.; voided 215 mL at 12:20 p.m.; voided 180 mL at 2:55 p.m.

Mother Teresa Care Center
Fluid Intake and Output Worksheet

Resident Name: _____   **Room:** _____

| Date | Time | Method of Adm | Intake | | | Output | | | |
			Solution	Amount	Time	Urine Amount	Other Output (specify)	Amount	Time

Developing Greater Insight

Answer the following questions based on this situation.

Mrs. Lebowitz is a 79-year-old cognitively impaired resident who does not speak. You have not cared for this resident in a week. The previous shift did not report any problems with the resident. She felt warm, so you checked her temperature. She has a fever of 99.8°F (O). She has been sleeping more than usual. She keeps falling asleep in her chair, which is out of character for the resident. She keeps rubbing her lower abdomen, which is slightly distended. She has had two small, incontinent, liquid stools today. This is unusual. You have been assigned to administer enemas to this resident before because she tends to be constipated. She has been passing gas. She has voided four times during the first four hours of your shift. Each time, she was incontinent a small amount of urine. Normally, she eats 100% of her meals, but today she is refusing to eat. She is taking liquids, but has complained of nausea. When you get the flow sheet book to document her liquid stools, you notice that she has not had a BM in three days. Four days ago she had a small BM. She had a small BM five days ago. She had no BM on day 6 or 7. She had a small BM on day 8. You see that her appetite has decreased over the past few days. This is the eighth day of the month, and the previous flow sheet is not in the book.

72. What action will you take?

_____

_____

73. What is the most likely cause of the resident's problem?

_____

_____

74. Why is liquid stool a sign of this problem?

_____

_____

75. Does this situation require immediate action, or will you report your observations at the end of the shift?

_____

_____

76. Document and total Mrs. Lebowitz's intake and output for your shift using the information below.

Intake				Output		
7:00	100 mL	water	PO	7:00	urinary drainage	200 mL
8:30	240 mL	tea	PO	11:00	vomitus	170 mL
10:30	120 mL	cranberry juice	PO	1:00	urinary drainage	150 mL
12:30	240 mL	broth	PO	1:45	vomitus	80 mL
2:00	100 mL	water	PO			
2:30	120 mL	sherbet	PO			

Mother Teresa Care Center
Fluid Intake and Output Worksheet

Resident Name: _____   Room: _____

Date	Time	Method of Adm	Intake			Output			
			Solution	Amount	Time	Urine Amount	Other Output (specify)	Amount	Time

77. Rearrange the letters to form a sentence in the lower grid. (Keep the letters in the same columns; skip a column for a space between words.)

S		O	T			G	B	R	E				A		
I	I	N	A		P	R	E	O	C	G		L	S	H	A	E	S	S
O	N	C	O	L	T	I	A	O	N	N	E	M	I	R	O	A	T	T	E
D	F	C	T	H	E	A	N	N	I	L	M	A	P	T	P	C	R	M	I

Hidden Picture

78. Carefully study the figure below and identify the barriers to aiding the resident's normal elimination pattern.

_____   _____   _____
_____   _____   _____
_____   _____   _____

CHAPTER 15

Restraints and Restraint Alternatives

KEY POINTS

- Restraints are safety devices.
- Restraints can be dangerous if used incorrectly or inappropriately.
- The least amount of restraint required to keep the resident safe should be used.
- Restraints may be used as enablers to empower the resident and improve independence.
- Risk factors in the environment should be eliminated to reduce the need for restraints.
- The use of alternatives to restraints should be considered and continually reevaluated.

ACTIVITIES

Vocabulary

Complete the puzzle by filling in the missing letters of words found in this chapter. Use the definitions to help you identify these words.

1. _ _ _ R _ _ _ _ _ RESTRAINT
2. _ E _ _ RESTRAINT
3. _ _ S _ RESTRAINT
4. _ _ _ T _ _
5. _ _ _ _ _ R _ _
6. _ _ _ _ _ _ A _ RESTRAINT
7. _ _ _ _ I _ _
8. _ N _ _ _ _ _
9. _ _ _ _ _ _ T
10. _ _ _ S _ _ _ _ RESTRAINT

1. a restraint used to secure an arm or leg
2. device that encircles the waist or hips to prevent sliding
3. applied to the upper body to prevent movement and sliding
4. farthest away from the center of the body
5. pertaining to body position
6. drugs used for discipline instead of medical problems
7. bending at a joint
8. device that helps resident to function independently
9. prop, bolster, position the resident to stabilize the body
10. device that restricts access to the body, restricts movement, and cannot be removed easily by the resident

True/False

Mark the following statements true or false.

11. T F Restraints should be used only as a last resort.
12. T F Restraints may be used for resident safety when the unit is short of staff.
13. T F Restraints may be used to keep wandering residents out of others' rooms.
14. T F Side rails may be safely left down when restraints are in use.
15. T F A device such as a sheet tucked in tightly is considered a restraint if the resident does not have the physical or mental ability to remove it easily.
16. T F Enablers are used to assist residents to function at their highest level.

17. T   F   Postural supports are restraints.
18. T   F   Restraints are applied according to manufacturers' directions.
19. T   F   Using restraints is the best way to prevent resident injuries.
20. T   F   "One size fits all" is a good rule of thumb to use when applying restraints.
21. T   F   The nursing assistant makes an important contribution to the restraint assessment.
22. T   F   Restraints can cause resident injuries and death.

Completion

Fill in the blanks to complete the chart. Identify each device as a restraint or restraint alternative based on the information listed.

Device	Restraint	Restraint Alternative
23. wheelchair lap tray secured with Velcro for a confused resident who has limited use of his arms		
24. vest applied to a resident who leans forward and falls each time she tries to stand unassisted		
25. fastening the wheelchair wheel to the hand rail in the hallway with a gait belt to prevent the wheelchair from moving		
26. tucking a sheet in loosely to cover a resident's lap for modesty when she is wearing a dress		
27. applying a belt to keep the resident in bed		
28. raising the side rails so the resident can pull on them and turn himself		
29. threading a sheet between the resident's legs, then tying it to the back of the chair to prevent her from sliding forward		
30. applying a belt with a Velcro fastener to a resident who needs a reminder to call for help		
31. applying a pressure-sensitive alarm when a resident is sitting up in a chair		
32. placing a piece of gripper under the resident to prevent her from sliding forward in the chair		

Complete the following statements by selecting the correct term from the list provided here.

alarm	environment	hips	reclining	ten
alignment	exercise	least	safety	thirty
armrest	feet	lock	seat	two
bathroom	fifteen	lowest	slip	unable
brakes	flexion	medical	small	under
chair	forward	movable	space	weight
entrapment	frame	over	springs	

33. When applying a vest to a resident in a wheelchair, thread the straps between the _____ and the _____ to keep the resident's _____ down.

34. Restraints must be released at least every _____ hours for at least _____ minutes.

35. Visually check the resident in restraints every _____ to _____ minutes.

36. Restraints must always be tied in a _____ knot.

37. The _____ restrictive restraint is used to keep the resident safe.

38. Consider the resident's _____ when selecting the restraint size.

39. Restraints are applied _____ the resident's clothing.

40. After applying a restraint, insert your fingers _____ the device to make sure it is not too tight.

41. The resident should be positioned in good _____ when restraints are used.

42. When a resident is restrained in a wheelchair, always _____ the _____ when the chair is parked.

43. Restraints are tied to the _____ of the wheelchair.

44. When a resident in a wheelchair is parked, the _____ front wheels should face _____.

45. Assist the resident to _____ and use the _____ when the restraint is released.

46. When the resident is in bed, fasten the restraint to the _____ part of the bed frame.

47. Tie the straps where the resident is _____ to reach them.

48. When the resident is in bed, the vest restraint should be tied to the bed _____, not the _____.

49. When applying an extremity restraint, position the extremity in a position of _____.

50. Using a _____ chair unnecessarily may cause the resident to lose touch with the _____.

51. Restraints are _____ devices.

52. Some restraint alternatives sound an _____ when the resident needs immediate assistance.

53. Always support the _____ when the resident is seated in a _____.

54. Restraints cannot be used without a valid, documented _____ reason.

55. The _____ between the side rail and the mattress should not be large enough to cause _____.

56. Keep the bed in the _____ possible position when the resident is in bed.

Developing Greater Insight

Answer the following questions based on this situation.

> Mrs. Libner is a mentally alert resident with a neurological condition that makes it difficult for her to sit upright and control her torso. Unsupported, she cannot maintain an upright position at meals and will fall over to the side of her chair. This increases her risk of choking and aspiration. She is unable to stand up and is dependent on staff for transfers. Various alternatives have been tried. The most successful is a Y- shaped shoulder harness similar to those the flight attendants wear on airplanes. A strap goes over each shoulder and connects to a special lap belt in front. The device is applied when she goes to the dining room. The harness and lap belt are removed when she leaves the room. She has lateral body support cushions on her chair to prevent injury. She occasionally falls to one side and must be repositioned, but the cushions prevent injury.

57. Is the Y-shaped shoulder harness a restraint or an enabler? Explain your answer.

_____

58. Are the lateral body support cushions restraints or enablers? Explain your answer.

_____

59. Would a vest restraint be more beneficial to this resident? Why or why not?

_____

60. Would this resident benefit from a pressure-sensitive alarm on the chair seat? Why or why not?

_____

Mrs. McCreedy was unsteady on her feet and at high risk of falls and other injuries. She began experiencing skin injuries and falls shortly after admission. She was placed in an adult walker, but she promptly tipped it. Restraining the resident in a wheelchair was ineffective, so the staff let her walk around and tried to watch her as best they could. She used a vest restraint when she was in bed. Despite the restraint, she was agitated and managed to get out of bed a number of times. Staff always made sure the side rails were raised to keep her safe. The resident's agitation worsened markedly and she was found to have a urinary tract infection. After treatment for infection, the agitation subsided to the resident's normal level. Mrs. McCreedy's pattern of falls with skin injuries persisted. She frequently fell on the way to the bathroom. She experienced 27 falls in $2\frac{1}{2}$ months. Although she fell frequently, the only injuries she sustained were bruises, scrapes, and skin tears. The nurse said they would look at the fall risk in the next care conference, which would be held in two weeks. The following day, Mrs. McCreedy was found on the floor with signs and symptoms of a hip fracture. Her left leg was shortened and rotated outward, and she was having severe pain. She was sent to the hospital where she was diagnosed with a hip fracture. She was admitted to the hospital, and surgery to repair the hip was scheduled for the next day.

61. Can you suggest at least one restraint alternative that should have been tried to keep this resident safe when she was up during the day? State why you think this device may have been effective for the resident.

_____

62. The resident's behavior worsened when she had an infection, and subsided when the infection was treated. Why is this useful to know? How will you use this information?

_____

_____

63. You are asked to participate in the resident's care conference. Mrs. McCreedy often fell while she was on the way to the bathroom. What information can you contribute to the care plan or suggest to reduce the risk of falls while on the way to the bathroom?

_____

_____

64. The vest restraint was discontinued when the resident returned from the hospital. The nurse asks your opinion on using the side rails during the care conference. Do the rails help keep this resident safe? Do the bed rails increase or decrease her risk of injury? Why or why not?

_____

_____

65. List three restraint alternatives that may be useful to prevent injury to the resident when she is in bed.

_____

_____

_____

66. Considering this resident's outcomes (27 falls, skin tears, bruises, abrasions, hip fracture), did the facility do a good job in keeping her safe? Why or why not?

_____

_____

67. In your opinion, did the facility meet the standard of care for this resident's safety? Explain your answer.

_____

_____

CHAPTER 16

Measuring Vital Signs, Height, and Weight

KEY POINTS

- Vital signs tell you how well the body's vital organs are working.

- Body temperature can be measured orally, rectally, at the axilla, or at the tympanic membrane.

- The site used most often for taking the pulse is the radial artery.

- Because respirations are under voluntary control, the resident should not know when you are counting them.

- The systolic blood pressure is the first sound heard when the heart is contracting.

- The diastolic blood pressure is the last sound heard when the heart is resting.

- Abnormal vital signs must be reported to the nurse immediately.

- Accuracy is very important when taking and recording vital signs.

- The nursing assistant is responsible for obtaining and accurately recording the resident's height and weight.

ACTIVITIES

Vocabulary

Complete the puzzle by filling in the missing letters of words found in this chapter. Use the definitions to help you identify these words.

1. _ _ _ H _ _ _ _ _ _ _
2. _ Y _ _ _ _ _
3. _ _ P _ _ _ _ _ _ _
4. _ _ _ _ _ E _
5. _ R _ _ _ _ _
6. _ _ _ T _ _ _ _
7. _ _ _ E _ _ _ _ _ _
8. _ _ _ _ _ _ _ N _ _ _ _ _ _
9. S _ _ _ _
10. _ _ _ _ _ I _
11. _ _ _ _ _ _ _ O _ _
12. _ N _ _ _ _ _

1. rapid pulse rate over 100 beats per minute
2. dark bluish or purplish color of skin and mucous membranes caused by inadequate oxygen
3. low blood pressure
4. felt
5. artery used for taking blood pressure
6. highest blood pressure reading
7. space in which the stethoscope is placed when taking blood pressure
8. blood pressure cuff and gauge
9. a surgically implanted passage between two blood vessels
10. lowest blood pressure reading
11. instrument used to hear body sounds
12. the spring-loaded dial marked with numbers to display the blood pressure reading

Completion

Fill in the blanks to complete the chart.

Your facility is having a flu epidemic. You have been assigned to take vital signs on C-wing. The tympanic thermometer was dropped earlier in the day and is broken. You will be using an electronic thermometer. The Director of Nursing's policy is that axillary temperatures are not to be taken except as a last resort, because they are the least accurate method of taking the temperature. Note the method you will use to take the temperature based on the information available.

The Resident	Oral Temperature	Rectal Temperature
13. has diarrhea		
14. is short of breath		
15. may have a fecal impaction		
16. is weak		
17. has a colostomy		
18. uses oxygen PRN; is not using it now		
19. is not responsive		
20. has been gagging and vomiting		
21. is alert and talks constantly		
22. has hemorrhoids		
23. is combative		
24. just returned to the facility after having prostate surgery		
25. is disoriented today, but follows instructions		
26. is coughing		
27. cannot breathe through the nose		
28. has a sore throat		

Complete the following statements by selecting the correct term from the list provided here.

2.5	diastolic	heart	oral	systolic
anus	dyspnea	heat	paralysis	tachycardia
apnea	exhalation	height	prehypertension	temperature
axillary	expansion	hypertension	probe cover	three
bradycardia	Fahrenheit	hypothermia	radial	thumb
Celsius	fifty	inhalation	rate	two
Cheyne-Stokes	force	mercury	rectal	tympanic
contraction	function	one	rhythm	weight

29. Vital signs are an indication of body _____.

30. Measurement of _____ is an indication of _____ in the body.

31. The pulse is a measurement of the heart _____.

32. The pulse is checked by feeling the _____ and _____ of an artery.

33. The blood pressure is a measurement of how hard the _____ is working.

34. Temperature is measured by using either a _____ or _____ scale.

35. The _____ of the pulse is an indication of how regularly the heart is beating.

36. Pulse rates lower than 60 beats per minute are called _____.

37. The _____ of the pulse is the strength of the beat.

38. _____ is the act of taking in air; _____ is the act of expelling air from the lungs.

39. Labored respirations and difficult breathing are called _____.

40. _____ respirations are often seen in a dying resident.

41. The medical term that means "no respirations" is _____.

42. You hear the _____ blood pressure during the working phase of the heart cycle.

43. You hear the _____ blood pressure when the heart is resting.

44. _____ is abnormally low body temperature (below 95°F).

45. Products containing _____ can be very toxic to humans and wildlife, if broken.

46. The _____ thermometer is used for taking the temperature in the inner ear.

47. When using the electronic thermometer, always cover the probe with a disposable _____.

48. The thermometer marked with a red tip is for taking a/an _____ temperature.

49. The thermometer marked with a blue tip is for taking a/an _____ temperature.

50. _____ is a blood pressure reading between 120/80 mm Hg and 139/89 mm Hg.

51. Do not take a blood pressure on an arm with _____, or inability to move.

52. The medical term for a pulse above 100 beats per minute is _____.

53. A blood pressure of 166/98 indicates a condition called _____.

54. The _____ is one indication of the resident's nutritional state.

55. The blood pressure cuff is positioned at least _____ inch above the elbow.

56. The lower bar on the standing balance scale is marked with lines every _____ pounds.

57. Even numbers are marked on the upper bar of the standing balance scale every _____ pounds.

58. One inch equals _____ centimeters.

59. The rectal temperature is taken by inserting the thermometer into the resident's _____.

60. The _____ temperature is taken by placing the thermometer under the arm.

61. The _____ pulse is located on the _____ side of the wrist.

62. When using a glass thermometer to measure oral or rectal temperature, leave the thermometer in place for at least _____ minutes.

63. The resident's _____ must be accurately measured on admission so the dietitian can determine the resident's normal body weight range.

Identification

Identify the equipment pictured.

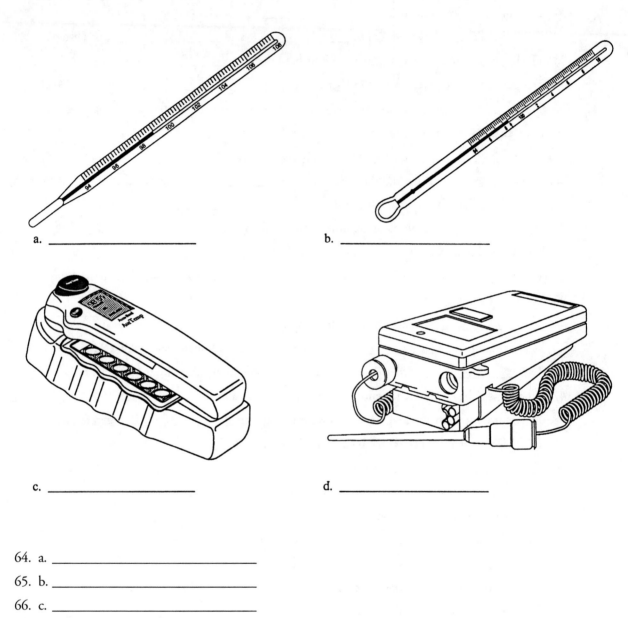

a. _____

b. _____

c. _____

d. _____

64. a. _____

65. b. _____

66. c. _____

67. d. _____

68. Refer to the figure below. Identify each thermometer (O = oral; R = rectal). Indicate the temperature reading.

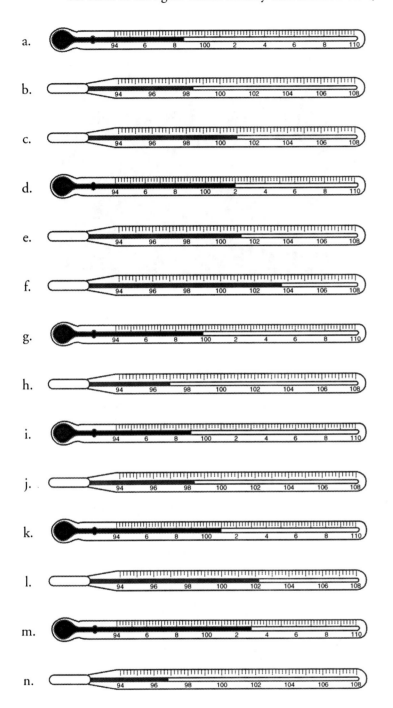

Type of thermometer	Reading
a. _____	_____
b. _____	_____
c. _____	_____
d. _____	_____
e. _____	_____
f. _____	_____
g. _____	_____
h. _____	_____
i. _____	_____
j. _____	_____
k. _____	_____
l. _____	_____
m. _____	_____
n. _____	_____

69. Refer to the figures below. Identify each item by name. Name the specific parts.

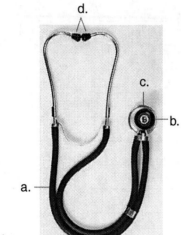

#1

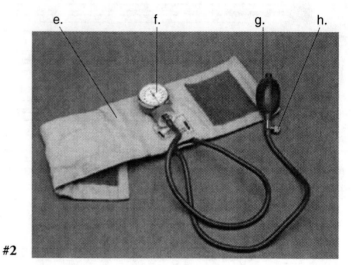

#2

Name of device #1: _____

    a. _____

    b. _____

    c. _____

    d. _____

Name of device #2: _____

    e. _____

    f. _____

    g. _____

    h. _____

70. Refer to the figures below. Determine the blood pressure values.

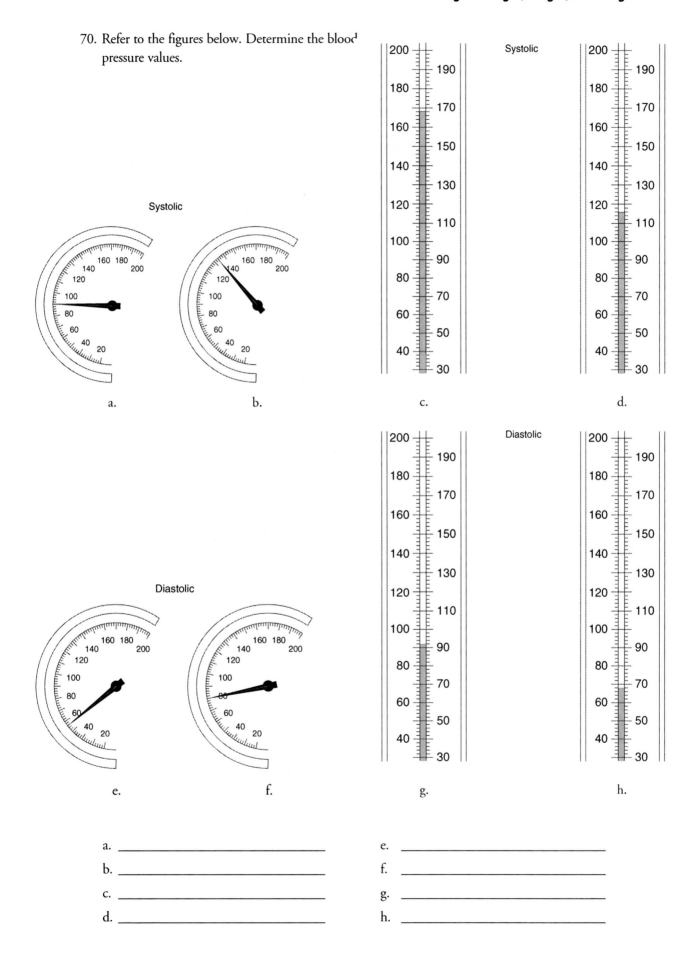

a. _____

b. _____

c. _____

d. _____

e. _____

f. _____

g. _____

h. _____

71. Refer to the figures below and on the following page. Read each scale and list the weight in the space provided.

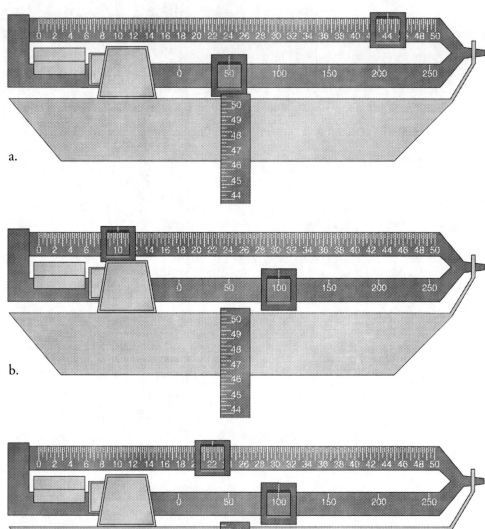

a.

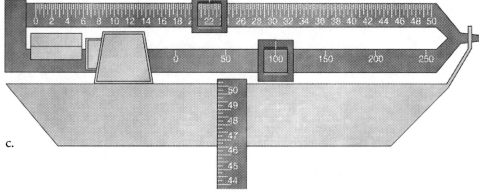

b.

c.

a. _____   d. _____

b. _____   e. _____

c. _____   f. _____

g. _____

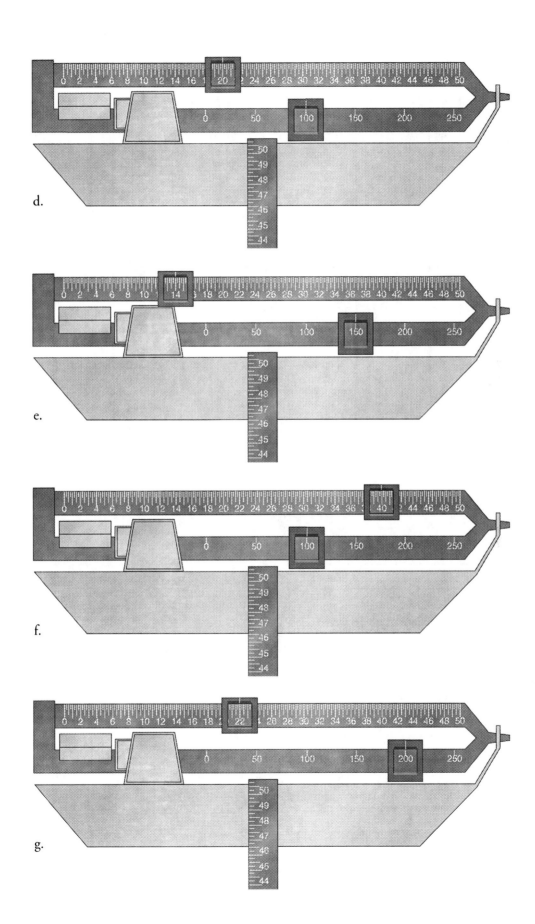

d.

e.

f.

g.

72. Refer to the figure below. Read each height measurement and document it in feet and inches in the space provided.

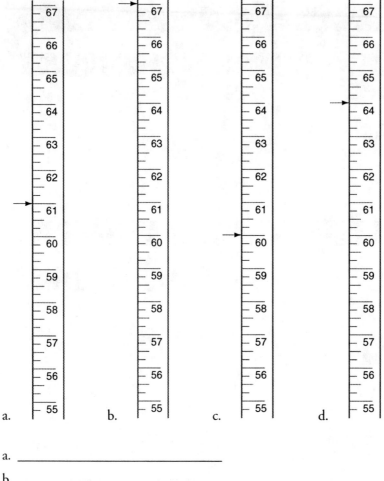

a.   b.   c.   d.

a. _____

b. _____

c. _____

d. _____

Developing Greater Insight

In your facility, a regular pulse may be counted for 30 seconds. Each of these pulses were counted for 30 seconds. What pulse rate will you record?

Counted Pulse   Recorded Pulse

73. 30 _____

74. 46 _____

75. 42 _____

76. 38 _____

77. 35 _____

78. 37 _____

79. 45 _____

80. 49 _____

Your facility policy requires a recheck of abnormal vital signs every four hours. Which of the following vital signs will you recheck? Which will you report to the nurse immediately?

	Vital Signs	Recheck in 4 Hours	Immediate Reporting
81.	98.2 (O) - 116-22-104/58		
82.	98.2 (O) - 88 -18-122/74		
83.	103.8 (R) -100-20-114/66		
84.	101.6 (O) - 74-16-124/82		
85.	99.4 (R) - 66-16-136/88		
86.	95.8 (O) - 100-20-110/60		
87.	99.0 (O) - 78-16-128/84		
88.	102.2 (R) - 60-14-112/64		
89.	100.6 (O) - 84-16-188/122		
90.	101.8 (R) - 92-20-142/104		

91. Rearrange the letters to form a sentence in the lower grid. (Keep the letters in the same columns; skip a column for a space between words.)

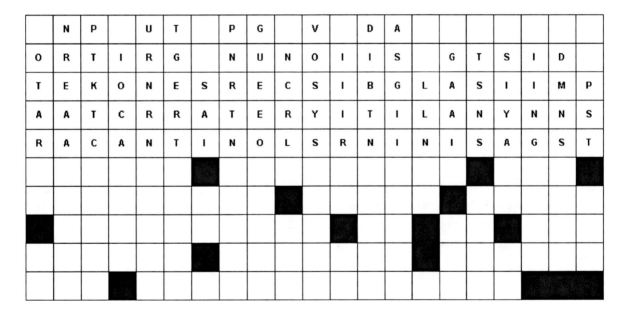

CHAPTER 17

Admission, Transfer, and Discharge

KEY POINTS

- The first impression that the resident has of the health care agency and its workers is a lasting one.

- The resident's perception of the admission process may be clouded by pain, illness, and fear.

- The nursing assistant is responsible for admitting the resident, gathering information, and making the resident comfortable.

- The nursing process involves assessment, planning, implementation, and evaluation.

- The nursing assistant makes valuable contributions to the nursing process.

- The nursing assistant is responsible for transferring the resident to a new unit within the health care facility, and ensuring the resident's comfort before leaving the unit.

- A physician's order is required for discharge from the health care facility.

- The nursing assistant is responsible for gathering the resident's belongings and safely escorting the resident to the car.

ACTIVITIES

Vocabulary

1. Complete the crossword puzzle.

Across

1 Family members are an _____ of the resident.

2 The social worker may also be called the discharge _____. He or she helps the resident make the transition when the resident returns to living in the community.

4 the procedure for helping the resident to leave the health care facility

8 the process of carrying out a plan

10 An IV _____ is a metal pole used to hang an IV bag, bottle, or pump above the infusion site.

11 moving the resident from one place, unit, or facility to another

12 gather information and facts to identify the resident's problems and needs

Down

1 The _____ services department is responsible for cleanliness and sanitation in most health care agencies.

3 the determination of how the resident's plan of care is working

5 the procedure that involves checking the resident into the facility and getting settled

6 deciding what to do with information gathered in an assessment

7 A professional demeanor and good _____ skills will help make the resident's admission a positive experience.

9 The resident and family must make many _____ during the transition to the long-term care facility.

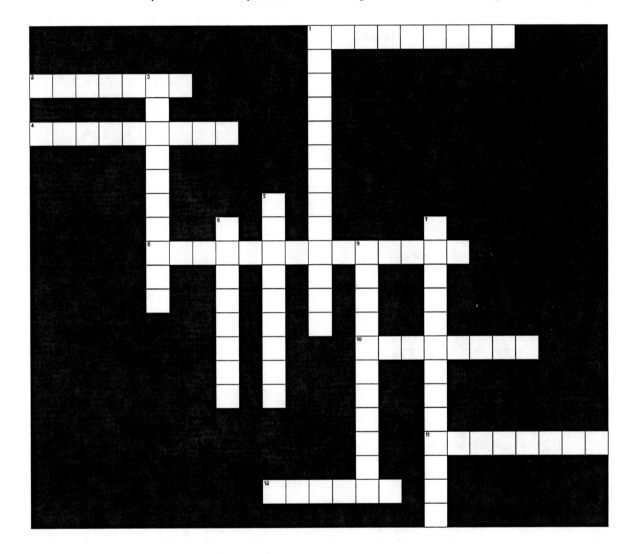

Completion

Complete the chart on admission activities. Indicate which activities are the nursing assistant's responsibility.

Activity	Nursing Assistant Responsibility	
	Yes	No
2. Check room to be sure it is ready for admission		
3. Explain advance directives to the resident and family		
4. Inform residents who are sharing the room with the new arrival		
5. Explain resident's rights		
6. Complete the clothing inventory		
7. Check the call signal and electric bed controls		
8. Check the bed for sheets, blanket, pillow, spread		
9. Make a complete assessment of the resident		
10. Make sure supplies such as an IV standard and trapeze are in the room		
11. Take the vital signs, height, and weight		
12. Check the closet for hangers		
13. Mark the resident's clothing (if needed) and put it away		
14. Observe the resident for visible problems and abnormalities		
15. Order medications from the pharmacy		
16. Make sure all the room lights are working		
17. Call the doctor and inform her of the admission		
18. Get the legal contracts signed and accept payment for the first month's stay		
19. Check to make sure the bathroom is clean before the resident arrives		
20. Place personal items and needed supplies in the bedside table		
21. Introduce yourself to the resident and family and explain your responsibilities in the care of the resident		
22. Introduce the new resident and family to roommates, if any		
23. Show the resident how to use the call signal		
24. Undress each new resident completely and assist him or her to bed		
25. Make the resident and family feel welcome; use good communication skills		
26. Read each of the admission papers sent from the hospital		
27. Determine the method of payment for services		
28. Tell the resident to provide a lock box, so valuables, money, and jewelry cannot be stolen		

True/False

Mark the following statements true or false.

29. T   F   First impressions are not usually important because the resident will see things differently after she adjusts to the facility.

30. T   F   The nursing assistant should strive to make the new resident's family feel welcome and comfortable.

31. T   F   When a resident is transferred to another room, all the personal belongings are also moved with the resident.

32. T   F   When transferring a resident, the nursing assistant should introduce the resident to staff on the new unit.

33. T   F   Discharge planning begins at the time of admission.

34. T   F   The nursing assistant does not contribute to the nursing assessment of the newly admitted resident; this is the nurses' responsibility.

35. T   F   The nursing assistant must make sure the resident is appropriately dressed at the time of discharge.

36. T   F   Admission to the long-term care facility is often an emotional time for the resident and family.

37. T   F   Family members should not assist with the resident's care.

38. T   F   Only licensed personnel are responsible for teaching and reinforcing residents' skills they will need after discharge.

39. T   F   Avoid addressing new residents by their first names without their permission.

40. T   F   The resident may leave the facility at any time; no physician order is necessary.

41. T   F   The nursing assistant is not responsible for transferring the resident's chart to the new unit in the facility.

42. T   F   Avoid speaking with family members during the admission process. This is the nurses' responsibility.

43. T   F   Do not leave the newly admitted resident's room until you have shown the resident how to use the call signal.

44. T   F   Most new residents are NPO until laboratory work is done.

45. T   F   If a resident's needs change, he or she may be transferred to a different unit or facility.

46. T   F   If a resident is transferred to the hospital for acute illness, you should protect valuables and put away items left in the room.

47. T   F   Nursing assistants are responsible for overall cleanliness and sanitation in the long-term care facility.

48. T   F   When a resident is discharged, family members are responsible for escorting him or her to the car.

49. T   F   The resident's perception of the admission process may be clouded by pain, illness, and fear.

50. T   F   The nursing assistant procedure for transferring a resident to another facility is usually similar to discharging the resident to home.

51. T   F   After a resident has been discharged, the nursing assistant should strip the unit.

Completion

A discharge checklist helps staff remember to complete their responsibilities. Complete the following checklist by listing at least eight additional nursing assistant responsibilities.

52.

	Discharge Checklist for: John S. Ardelean
	Initial Each Task After Completion

Initials	Nursing Assistant Responsibilities
SR	1. Follow facility policies and supervisors' instructions.
SR	2. Assist the resident to dress and gather belongings, as needed.
	3.
	4.
	5.
	6.
	7.
	8.
	9.
	10.

_____

Date and Time   Nursing Assistant Signature

Developing Greater Insight

Answer the following questions (53 to 56) based on these situations.

Mrs. Wolverton is being admitted to the skilled nursing unit of your facility after a long hospitalization. Prior to her illness, she lived alone in her home with her little dog. Her husband of 54 years died two years ago. The resident is fragile in appearance, weak, and tired. However, she is mentally alert, pleasant, and polite. She confides in you that she feels bad that she must accept charity help from the Medicare program, which is covering her stay. She gets tears in her eyes when she tells you that her little dog is being cared for by her daughter.

53. What losses do you think the resident has suffered and how have these affected her?

_____

_____

54. Do you think the resident is comfortable with her financial situation?

_____

55. Do you think anxiety will make admission more difficult for the resident?

_____

56. What can the nursing assistant do to make the transition to facility living easier for the resident?

_____

_____

Mrs. Brasa is being admitted to your facility. She is sitting in a wheelchair, holding her daughter's hand tightly. She is tearful and obviously fearful. The daughter also appears anxious. You show her how to use the call signal, but she says she is afraid no one will come if she needs help.

57. How can you reassure this resident that staff will respond if she signals?

_____

_____

58. What can the nursing assistant do to ease the resident's anxiety?

_____

_____

59. Mrs. Brasa brought the following personal items with her to the facility: 19-inch color television with remote control, 7 pairs slacks, 8 blouses, 10 panties, 12 pairs socks, 2 sweatshirts, 2 sweat pants, 3 nightgowns, 1 robe, 1 pair slippers, 1 pair tennis shoes, 1 sweater, 1 jacket, 1 pink-and-white afghan, 1 clock radio, 1 pair eyeglasses, 1 hearing aid, upper dentures, lower partial plate, toothbrush, denture paste, 1 box denture tablets, denture cup, hairbrush, comb, 1 bottle lotion, 1 roll-on deodorant, 1 bottle cologne, 1 makeup kit, 1 curling iron, 4 family photos, 2 pink, heart-shaped throw pillows, 1 armchair with footstool, 1 black leather purse, 1 black leather wallet, 1 wristwatch, 4 pairs stud-type pierced earrings, gold necklace, gold bracelet, gold wedding ring. Complete the personal inventory record on page 132 by listing the resident's personal property.

INVENTORY OF PERSONAL EFFECTS
(Reference tag: F252)

INSTRUCTIONS: Upon admission, identify the resident's personal belongings by indicating quantity of those items listed. Use the space allowed to write in additional items as necessary. The original copy shall be kept in the resident's chart. The copy is given to the resident or resident representative. Update as necessary throughout the resident's stay by using the space provided. Upon discharge, use the "√" columns to indicate that all personal belongings are accounted for.

QTY.	ARTICLES	√
	Belts	
	Blouses	
	Coats	
	Dresses	
	Gloves	
	Handkerchiefs	
	Hats	
	Housecoats/robes	
	Jackets	
	Nightgowns/pajamas	
	Purses	
	Shaving kit	
	Shoes	
	Shorts	
	Slacks	
	Slippers	
	Slips	
	Shirts	
	Socks/hose	
	Suitcases	
	Suits	
	Suspenders	
	Sweaters	
	Ties	
	Undershirts	
	Underwear	
	Hearing aid	
	Dentures: ☐ Up ☐ Low ☐ Part	
	Eyewear	
	Cane	
	Walker	
	Wheelchair	
	Brace	
	Prosthesis	

ITEMS OF SPECIFIC VALUE (JEWELRY, APPLIANCES, FURNITURE)

QTY	DESCRIPTION	VALUE	√
		$	

ITEMS ACQUIRED AFTER ORIGINAL ENTRY

DATE	ITEM	HOW RECEIVED	INITIAL	√

USE THIS SPACE TO RECORD MISCELLANEOUS INFORMATION (i.e. LOST, STOLEN, RETURNED/GIVEN TO FAMILY, ETC.)

DATE	DESCRIPTION / EXPLANATION	INITIAL	√

CERTIFICATION OF RECEIPT

ON ADMISSION

Signed X _____ Date _____
Resident or resident representative

Signed _____ Title _____ Date _____
Facility representative

If resident unable to sign, state reason:

Signed _____ Date _____
Witness

ON DISCHARGE

Signed X _____ Date _____
Resident or resident representative

Signed _____ Title _____ Date _____
Facility representative

If resident unable to sign, state reason:

Signed _____ Date _____
Witness

NAME—Last	First	Middle	Attending Physician	Chart No.

CFS 1-12/2P © 1992 Briggs Corporation, Des Moines, IA 50306 (800) 247-2343
R1096   Printed in U.S.A.

INVENTORY OF PERSONAL EFFECTS

60. Rearrange the letters to form a sentence in the lower grid. (Keep the letters in the same columns; skip a column for a space between words.)

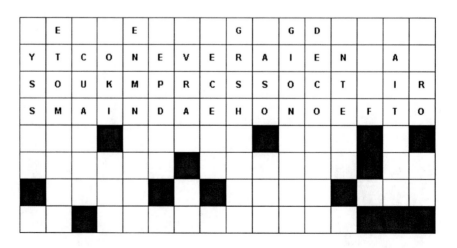

CHAPTER 18

Restorative Care

KEY POINTS

- Restorative care is given to assist residents to attain and maintain their highest level of function.

- Promoting independence is part of restorative care.

- Restorative care is most effective if it is started early in the resident's illness.

- Activity strengthens residents and inactivity weakens.

- When providing restorative care, stress what the resident can do.

- When providing restorative care, the nursing assistant should look at the entire person and not just the illness.

- Many restorative programs involve assisting residents to relearn ADL skills.

- Range of motion is normal movement of joints.

- If a resident's joints do not move through the normal range of motion each day, contractures and deformities may develop.

- Contractures promote pressure ulcer development, and make treating pressure ulcers more difficult.

- Residents with existing contractures are at high risk of developing additional contractures. Contractures can begin to develop in as little as four days of immobility and inactivity. After 15 days, the resident will lose range of motion.

- Arthritis can cause mild discomfort to severe deformities and disability; the most common symptom is pain.

- Osteoporosis is a metabolic disorder in which bone mass is lost, causing bones to become porous and spongy. Residents with this condition are at very high risk for fractures.

- Hip fracture is the most common fracture in the elderly. The term "hip fracture" refers to a fracture anywhere in the upper third or head of the femur.

- A cerebrovascular accident is caused by a sudden interruption of blood to the brain. Residents with this condition will experience weakness or paralysis on one side of the body; other complications such as speech and vision problems may also occur.

- A transient ischemic attack is a temporary period of diminished blood flow to the brain that occurs suddenly and usually lasts from 2 to 15 minutes. Residents with this condition are at risk of stroke.

- Parkinson's disease is an incurable neurological disease that causes tremors and shuffling gait, and increases the risk of injury.

- Huntington's disease is an incurable neurological disease that is hereditary. The resident develops choreiform movements, loss of voluntary movement, and dementia.

- Multiple sclerosis is a progressive neurological disorder that causes a degeneration of the nervous system and interferes with conduction of nerve impulses.

- Post polio syndrome is a neurologic condition marked by increased weakness and abnormal muscle fatigue in persons who had polio many years earlier. Estimates are that 30% to 70% of all polio survivors will develop this condition.

- Head injuries usually result from trauma, falls, or automobile accidents. The injury often causes severe, permanent brain damage. Residents with brain injury are often totally dependent on staff for care.

- Spinal cord injuries commonly cause paralysis that affects sensation and voluntary movement below the level of injury.

- A self-care deficit is an inability to perform an activity of daily living.

- Bowel and bladder retraining programs are individualized to the resident's needs based on an assessment.

- Kegel exercises strengthen pelvic floor muscles, and the muscles surrounding the urethra and vagina; they are helpful in preventing incontinence.

- Trochanter rolls should be used routinely for bedfast residents to prevent deformities caused by external rotation of the hip.

- The nursing assistant is responsible for applying and removing many types of restorative equipment.

ACTIVITIES

Vocabulary

Fit the words into the puzzle on page 136. Define each term.

4 letters

1. CUES _____

5 letters

2. KEGEL _____

3. RANGE _____

6 letters

4. FLEXION _____

5. MEDIAL _____

7 letters

6. ATROPHY _____

7. BEDREST _____

8. DEFICIT _____

9. SPLINTS _____

8 letters

10. ADAPTIVE _____

11. EVERSION _____

12. MOBILITY _____

13. ORTHOTIC _____

14. ROTATION _____

9 letters

15. ABDUCTION _____

16. ADDUCTION _____

17. DEPENDENT _____

18. EXTENSION _____

19. INVERSION _____

20. POSTPOLIO _____

10 letters

21. AUTOIMMUNE _____

22. HEMIPLEGIA _____

23. IMMOBILITY _____

24. INACTIVITY _____

25. OPPOSITION _____

26. PARKINSONS _____

27. PROSTHESIS _____

28. SPASTICITY _____

29. TROCHANTER _____

11 letters

30. HEMIPARESIS _____

31. HUNTINGTONS _____

32. RESTORATION _____

12 letters

33. CONTRACTURES _____

34. DORSIFLEXION _____

35. OSTEOPOROSIS _____

13 letters

36. CIRCUMDUCTION _____

37. EXACERBATIONS _____

14 letters

38. HYPEREXTENSION _____

39. REHABILITATION _____

15 letters

40. CEREBROVASCULAR _____

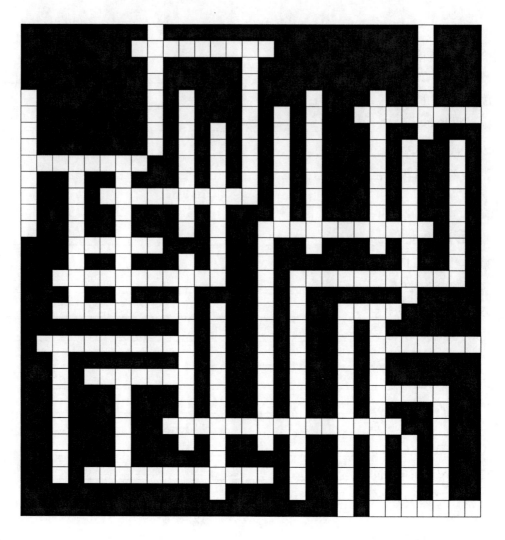

True/False

Mark the following statements true or false.

41. T F   Pressure ulcers may worsen rapidly and be difficult or impossible to reverse.

42. T F   The term *hip fracture* refers to a fracture anywhere in the lower half of the femur.

43. T F   Residents with post polio syndrome have severe cold intolerance, even with mild cold exposure.

44. T F   Residents with Parkinson's disease walk with stiff, spastic movements.

45. T F   Contractures promote pressure ulcer development.

46. T F   Huntington's disease can be cured if diagnosed early.

47. T F   Residents who have had hip surgery use an adduction pillow postoperatively.

48. T F   Residents with Huntington's disease usually gain weight because of inactivity.

49. T F   Contractures cause reduced capillary blood flow to bony prominences.

50. T F   Hip fractures are the most common fractures in the elderly.

51. T F   Most polio survivors are fiercely independent.

52. T F   Signs and symptoms of a TIA are similar to those of a heart attack.

53. T F   Paralysis affects sensation and voluntary movement above the level of injury.

54. T F   The most common symptom of arthritis is spasticity.

55. T F   Residents who have severe brain damage are able to open their eyes, but seem unaware or minimally aware of their surroundings.

56. T F A resident with a neurogenic bladder has frequent urges to use the bathroom.

57. T F The trochanter roll is used to prevent internal rotation of the hips.

58. T F Residents with arthritis are at high risk of contractures.

59. T F Kegel exercises help prevent incontinence.

60. T F Abnormal movements, called chorea, are the primary sign of multiple sclerosis.

61. T F Fractures can occur spontaneously in residents with osteoporosis, such as when turning the resident over in bed.

62. T F Stress, infection, and injury may trigger remissions in multiple sclerosis.

63. T F Contractures begin to develop after about four months of immobility and inactivity.

64. T F Every muscle has an antagonist that works in the opposite direction.

65. T F Residents who have had hip surgery are at very high risk of developing heel pressure ulcers.

Identification

66. Identify each joint action.

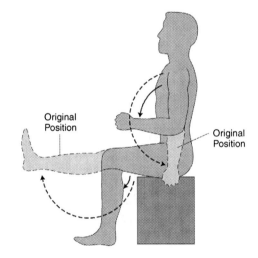

a. _____

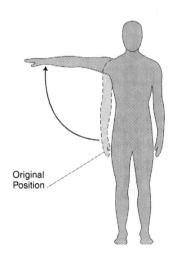

b. _____

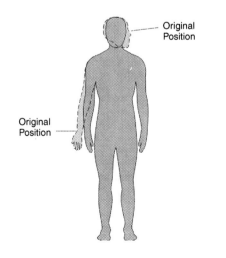

c. _____

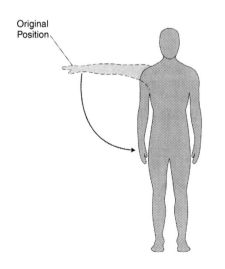

d. _____

Completion

Place an X in the box to determine appropriate or inappropriate nursing assistant actions. If the action is inappropriate, write the appropriate action in the space provided. One example is provided.

Action	Appropriate	Inappropriate	Alternate Action
Unlock the wheels to the bed before beginning range-of-motion exercises.		X	lock the wheels
67. Raise the bed to a comfortable working height before beginning range-of-motion exercises.			
68. Give restorative care a purpose, whenever possible, such as walking back and forth in the hallway.			
69. Encourage independence for alert residents and dependence for confused residents.			
70. If a resident does not respond to verbal cues, finish the task for the resident.			
71. Sincerely compliment the resident for the part of the task she was able to complete.			
72. If the resident complains of pain during range of motion, stop the activity.			
73. Prevent pressure ulcers on the heels by applying heel protectors to bedfast residents.			
74. Monitor the pulse during range of motion. Stop the activity if the pulse exceeds 92.			
75. If a resident is rigid, do range-of-motion exercises in the shower or whirlpool.			
76. Schedule a time that is convenient for you to assist each resident with restorative care.			
77. Assist residents on bowel and bladder retraining programs to use the bathroom every two hours, without exception.			

Developing Greater Insight

Answer the following questions based on this situation.

Mr. Ng is a 48-year-old resident who was admitted because his legs were crushed in an industrial accident, in which he was pinned against the wall by a forklift. The injuries were severe, and the resident experienced infection and other complications. The legs could not be saved and both legs were amputated above the knee. He plans to return home to his wife and teenage son when he becomes more independent. He tells you he used to coach his son's softball team, and really misses it. His son's picture is on the dresser, and you know the son is a source of great pride for the resident. The resident is making good progress in learning to use prosthetic legs in therapy. He has had some problems with raw skin areas under the prostheses. He frequently complains of phantom pain, and is easily frustrated.

78. Mr. Ng is frustrated this morning. He admits he is anxious to go home. His "left foot" is very painful. He says his progress is "just too slow." Breakfast is in an hour, and he asks to stay in bed. You know he has therapy immediately after breakfast, and must be up. It takes about 30 minutes to get the resident up, washed, and dressed, and you have other residents to get up and feed. You know the therapy is important if the resident wants to return home soon. How can a nursing assistant handle this situation? Describe the highest priority that you will address first. Then state other actions you will take to meet the resident's needs.

_____

_____

_____

_____

_____

_____

79. Rearrange the letters to form two sentences in the lower grid. (Keep the letters in the same columns; skip a column for a space between words.)

	H	W		I			B	B		L	S	Y			H	N		R	O	T	
D	L	E	A	D	I	E	A	T	L	I	T	D		A	N	D		M	O	S	E
T	E	N	S	Y	S	A	N	I	I	I	I	T	Y	P	E	R	D	N	N	T	E
A	R	E	T	S	D	S	S	T	R	E	N	S	E	T	P	E	O	E	E	C	I
						■							■				■				
					■										■		■				■
			■											■							
■							■														

CHAPTER 19

The Nursing Assistant in Subacute Care

KEY POINTS

- Residents in the subacute unit have complex needs and their conditions can change very quickly.

- The nursing assistant in subacute care must have excellent technical and observational skills.

- The five types of subacute units are transitional, general medical-surgical, chronic subacute, long-term transitional subacute, and specialty subacute.

- Many residents in the subacute unit are monitored with a pulse oximeter to measure the amount of oxygen in their arterial blood.

- A basic knowledge of sterile technique is necessary for the nursing assistant working in the subacute care unit.

ACTIVITIES

Vocabulary

Match the terms on the right with the definitions on the left.

1. _____ cancer treatment that employs specific chemical agents to destroy cancer cells

2. _____ device that measures the oxygen in the arterial blood

3. _____ method of connecting an artery and vein with a tube for use in dialysis

4. _____ plastic or metal tube inserted into a tracheostomy to keep the stoma open

5. _____ opening into the trachea through which the resident breathes

6. _____ a portable form of dialysis performed in subacute care centers

7. _____ site where the intravenous needle is inserted into the body

8. _____ cancer treatment in which the skin is exposed to high doses of radiation

9. _____ passage between two blood vessels, commonly used for dialysis

10. _____ clamp used to close tubes quickly

11. _____ abnormal heart rhythm

12. _____ removing waste products from the body by cleansing the resident's blood

13. _____ care given to residents after surgical procedures

14. _____ method of feeding total nutrition intravenously which allows the GI system to rest

15. _____ intravenous line inserted in the arm and threaded through the venous system to the superior vena cava

16. _____ device used to assist or control breathing

a. shunt
b. infusion site
c. hemodialysis
d. peripherally inserted central catheter
e. total parenteral nutrition
f. radiation therapy
g. pulse oximeter
h. dysrhythmia
i. graft
j. ventilator
k. cannula
l. chemotherapy
m. tracheostomy
n. Kelly
o. continuous ambulatory peritoneal dialysis
p. postoperative care

Completion

Complete the following statements by selecting the correct term from the list provided here.

70	chronic	fluid restriction	pathogen
above	contaminated	four	quickly
alarms	documentation	handling	shaving
alopecia	drainage	IV	three
below	eat	linen	toothbrush
chemotherapy	fatigue	long term transitional	tremors

17. Staff in the subacute unit must have good observational skills, because the residents' conditions can change _____.

18. The _____ subacute unit provides care for residents with complex medical needs or residents connected to ventilators.

19. When residents are receiving chemotherapy, their soiled _____ will probably require special _____.

20. _____ must reflect the resident's progress toward care plan goals and response to treatment.

21. Do not use an electronic blood pressure monitor to check blood pressure on a resident with _____.

22. If a resident has an implanted radiation device, stay at least _____ feet away from the resident unless direct care is being delivered.

23. The _____. subacute unit provides care for residents with little hope of recovery and return to functional independence.

24. Residents receiving chemotherapy will probably need a very soft _____.

25. If residents are connected to electronic devices for vital sign monitoring, respond to equipment _____ immediately.

26. Pulse oximeter finger sensors should be rotated at least every _____ hours.

27. Avoid taking blood pressure on the arm with an _____.

28. Sterile technique is a _____-free technique.

29. Residents receiving _____ may excrete the drugs in their waste and body fluids.

30. Common side effects of chemotherapy include _____ and _____.

31. Avoid _____ areas near the radiation treatment field.

32. Signs and symptoms of wound infection may include increased _____.

33. When you are wearing sterile gloves, keep your hands _____ your waist.

34. Pulse oximeter readings below _____ % indicate life-threatening conditions.

35. If a sterile item becomes wet, it is _____.

36. Never _____ in an area where chemotherapy is being prepared.

37. Never position a container of intravenous solution _____ the needle insertion site.

38. When a resident is receiving dialysis, the physician commonly orders a _____.

Completion

Complete the chart by indicating which activities are the nursing assistant's responsibility.

Activity	Nursing Assistant Responsibility	
	Yes	No
39. taking blood pressure with an electronic monitoring device		
40. administering chemotherapy		
41. monitoring for intravenous infiltration		
42. changing the flow rate of the intravenous solution		
43. observing and reporting the effects of chemotherapy drugs		
44. monitoring for signs and symptoms of infection		
45. assisting residents receiving chemotherapy with elimination		
46. marking the skin for radiation therapy after bathing the resident		
47. monitoring pulse oximeter values		
48. monitoring residents for pain		
49. disconnecting electronic monitoring devices so personal care can be given		
50. caring for the tracheostomy cannula		
51. positioning residents with serious wounds on a low air loss bed		
52. assisting with sterile procedures		
53. administering TPN		
54. adjusting the ventilator settings		
55. using the Kelly to clamp a broken PICC line		
56. monitoring residents who are receiving CAPD		
57. assisting with postoperative monitoring and care		
58. monitoring residents after dialysis		
59. changing the intravenous solution		
60. monitoring and documenting strict intake and output		

True/False

Mark the following statements true or false.

61. T   F   Residents needing subacute care stay in the skilled nursing unit.

62. T   F   Residents needing therapy services on the subacute unit usually receive three to five hours of therapy each day, so the nursing assistant must coordinate the timing of nursing care with therapy services.

63. T   F   A resident who is connected to a ventilator will be unable to speak.

64. T   F   Wash the tracheostomy stoma well with plenty of soap and water, pat dry with cotton.

65. T   F   Inform the nurse if a resident has foul-smelling wound drainage.

66. T   F   If the sterility of any item is in doubt, consider it unsterile.

67. T   F   If sterile items become wet, they may be used if they are on the sterile field.

68. T   F   The tips of the subclavian catheter and PICC line are threaded through the venous system to the upper chamber of the heart.

69. T   F   Air in the subclavian line can be fatal.

70. T   F   Pain in the neck and chest is normal when residents have a subclavian line.

71. T   F   Adjust the clamps on the intravenous tubing as needed to control the flow rate.

72. T   F   Disconnect the IV temporarily when changing the resident's gown, then reconnect it.

73. T   F   Force fluids for residents who are receiving dialysis.

74. T   F   Monitor dialysis residents for dizziness and hypotension.

75. T   F   When a resident is receiving CAPD, the dialysate that returns will appear slightly bloody.

76. T   F   Residents who are receiving hospice services and those with terminal AIDS are not good candidates for the subacute unit.

77. T   F   Chemotherapy drugs cannot differentiate cancer cells from normal cells, so other cells are also affected.

78. T   F   The risk of bleeding is increased when residents receive chemotherapy.

79. T   F   Residents who are receiving radiation and chemotherapy are often served low-protein meals and snacks.

80. T   F   Apply lotion to lubricate the radiation treatment field each day.

Developing Greater Insight

Answer the following questions based on this situation.

Mr. Zaugg is an alert resident who receives chemotherapy. He has been weak, and experiences pain, nausea, and vomiting. The inside of his mouth is sore, with some white patches and areas of bleeding on the gums. His appetite has been poor and he has lost weight. He has an order for daily weight monitoring. He receives six small meals a day, and has no special dietary restrictions. He has an order for supplements between meals, force fluids, and intake and output.

81. You take the resident's supper tray to the room. He looks at it and says he does not want it. He says he wishes he were at home, where he could make a baked potato with melted cheese for supper. He asks you to take the tray away. How can you assist this resident?

----

82. You bring a canned, liquid supplement to the resident's room. He says he does not like the flavor. He also says that the warm (room-temperature) supplement drinks make him gag. What action will you take?

----

83. Mr. Zaugg likes fruit juice. He receives a variety of juices on his trays each day. Orange juice is his favorite. Although the resident has an order to force fluids, he says the juice hurts his mouth too much, so he does not drink it. The nurse informed you in report that his lab reports reveal he is becoming dehydrated. How can you assist this resident with his fluid intake?

_____

_____

84. Mr. Zaugg's fluid intake was 1,050 mL at the end of the day shift on Tuesday. When you pick up the I&O worksheets on Wednesday, his total fluid intake for day shift is listed as 165 mL. What action will you take first? What will you do next?

_____

_____

CHAPTER 20

Special Behavioral Problems

KEY POINTS

- All behavior has a meaning, even if the meaning is not evident to you.
- Losses and unmet needs affect residents' behavior.
- Physical and chemical restraints are the treatment of last resort in the management of behavior problems.
- When using the ABC method of behavior management, modifying the antecedent or consequences will change the behavior.
- Consistency is important to the success of a behavior management program.
- Cognitive impairment has many causes, and is not a normal part of aging.
- Safety is a primary concern when caring for residents who have cognitive impairment and dementia.
- Delirium is a reversible condition with medical causes.
- Sensory losses may mimic cognitive impairment or worsen existing dementia.
- Alzheimer's disease causes atrophy of the brain and progressive mental deterioration.
- Wandering is a serious problem in long-term care facilities. The nursing assistant plays an important role in preventing the wanderer from leaving or becoming injured.

ACTIVITIES

Vocabulary

Each line has four different spellings of a word from this unit. Circle the correctly spelled word.

1. antesedant	antissedint	antecedent	anteseadent
2. catastrophic reaction	katastroffic reacshun	catistrophic reaxtion	catestrofic reaction
3. cognutife impearmant	cognitive impairment	cognative impairmint	cognatife impairmunt
4. combative behavior	commbative behafior	kombatife behaviore	cumbative behavore
5. compunsation	compunsashun	compensation	compinsation
6. consickwences	consiquensis	consaquenses	consequences
7. cunsistant	consistent	consistant	kansistent
8. dillerium	dilyreum	dellereum	delirium
9. delusions of persecution	dillushuns of persicushun	dilutions of persicutune	delushuns of persicution
10. dimmensha	dementia	dimentia	damensha
11. dippresion	deppreshun	depression	dapresion
12. disoriented	disoreentid	desoriented	dissoreented
13. hullucinashuns	halucinasions	hulusinations	hallucinations
14. pirseferashun	perseveration	perrseverasion	purrseveration
15. projecshun	projecsion	projection	progection

16. rationalization	rashunalisation	racionalisashun	ratunalizatiun
17. reallity oreentation	realety oreintashun	realetty orientasion	reality orientation
18. reminiscing	remenissing	remminising	remoniscing
19. sensurry loss	sensory loss	sensorry loss	sencorry loss
20. sexule abuce	sexuale abuss	sexual abuse	sectual ebuss
21. sundowng	sundowning	sundowneng	sunndowning
22. validation therapy	falidasion tharapy	validashun tharepy	vallidasion therappy

Find the four defense mechanisms listed in the puzzle. Define each.

c	l	e	w	n	o	i	t	c	e	j	o	r	p	r
n	y	k	j	n	m	e	e	m	f	w	q	h	a	m
x	o	q	v	v	j	h	r	d	i	x	v	t	q	k
e	m	i	f	g	o	n	u	o	k	z	i	m	p	n
d	r	x	t	g	w	b	z	f	q	o	w	w	k	s
f	b	r	c	a	k	x	i	y	n	z	g	b	o	x
p	p	v	z	k	s	z	p	a	d	n	n	n	g	w
g	n	h	p	u	f	n	l	q	f	n	z	y	h	f
t	s	r	g	r	m	i	e	i	t	s	g	a	p	b
i	s	n	l	p	z	j	n	p	i	r	c	x	i	j
i	f	j	w	a	z	y	a	b	m	x	e	y	l	d
v	f	x	t	z	w	d	t	h	f	o	v	v	l	k
k	i	i	s	c	a	p	a	c	n	o	c	a	o	z
w	o	n	k	y	m	e	r	v	s	a	z	t	s	r
n	q	t	z	g	s	l	i	i	l	a	i	n	e	d

23. _____

24. _____

25. _____

26. _____

Completion

Complete the following statements by selecting the correct term from the list provided here.

abnormal behavior	defense	masturbation	rights
Alzheimer's Disease	dignity	meaning	self-care ability
bathroom	discouragement	modify	self-control
care plan	distract	overwhelmed	stress
communicating	front	reality orientation	sundowning
consent	harm	reason	thirsty
coping	identity	reminiscence	unmet needs
covering	losses	restraints	

27. Behavior problems are often the result of _____.

28. A confused resident may demonstrate behavior problems when she is _____ or needs to use the _____.

29. When managing behavior problems, _____ are a treatment of last resort.

30. Most long-term care facility residents have experienced many _____.

31. All behavior has a _____, even if you are not aware of it.

32. Residents use _____ and _____ mechanisms as tools to compensate for losses and as a response to _____.

33. Nursing assistants may need to _____ their behavior in response to the residents' behavior.

34. Residents with depression have feelings of despair and _____.

35. Always report _____ to the nurse, even if you believe the behavior is "normal for the resident."

36. If a resident is agitated, aggressive, and may strike out, always approach him or her from the _____.

37. _____ the elevator buttons with fabric or duct tape may keep wandering residents away from them.

38. When assisting residents with behavior problems, follow the approaches listed on the _____ in the order listed.

39. Validation helps residents regain feelings of _____ and _____.

40. Maintaining the _____ and dignity of residents is important.

41. _____ is most effective in orienting residents with delirium.

42 When using _____, you will assist residents to remember their past.

43. _____ is an acceptable behavior as long as it is done in a private area.

44. Adults have a legal right to do whatever is pleasing to them, as long as it is not medically contraindicated and both partners are mentally capable of _____.

45. Loss of _____ is often the first sign of cognitive impairment.

46. Residents who have dementia have the same _____ as other residents.

47. Residents who have sensory loss may have difficulty _____ with others.

48. _____ is the most common form of dementia.

49. Residents who have delusions of persecution fear others will _____ them.

50. Residents who are _____ commonly wander in the evening and at night.

51. A resident having a catastrophic reaction feels completely _____.

52. Residents with Alzheimer's disease lose the ability to _____.

53. You may be able to _____ a wandering resident with food or drink.

Completion

Write the information in the space provided.

54. Identify the three components of the ABC plan and describe how each is used.

_____

_____

_____

55. List at least 10 guidelines for managing behavior problems.

_____

_____

_____

_____

_____

_____

_____

_____

_____

_____

56. List at least five ways of assisting residents with depression.

_____

_____

_____

_____

57. List at least five ways of assisting residents with complaining or demanding behavior.

_____

_____

_____

_____

58. List at least 10 guidelines for assisting residents who display aggressive behavior.

_____

_____

_____

_____

_____

_____

_____

_____

59. List at least 10 guidelines for managing wandering behavior.

_____

_____

_____

_____

_____

_____

_____

_____

_____

Developing Greater Insight

Answer the following questions based on this situation.

You are working as a nursing assistant on the 3:00 p.m. to 11:00 p.m. shift at the Quality Care Convalescent Center. Dr. Zeleski is a 57-year-old resident with Alzheimer's disease. He was formerly a college professor. His hair is salt-and-pepper black and gray. He is a well-groomed, good-looking man with a dignified appearance who dresses in color-coordinated sweaters and casual slacks. Dr. Zeleski has good communication skills, and seems to be alert during a brief conversation. When you visit for longer periods of time, you realize he is very disoriented, and does not use good judgment. Because of his good communication skills, age, and appearance, he is often mistaken for a visitor in the facility. Dr. Zeleski's wife cared for him at home until she had a stroke and was hospitalized. She is in the subacute unit of the local hospital. The resident's daughter tried to care for the doctor in her home, but gave up after several days. The doctor left food unattended on the stove, and forgot the burners were on. He wandered outside in the middle of the night on several occasions. The temperature was very cold and he was not appropriately dressed. Fortunately, his daughter was a very light sleeper. She nailed long chains of loud jingle bells over the doors so that if he went outside, the bells would awaken her. Fortunately, this approach was successful, but having him in the house was very stressful for the daughter's family.

Because of the resident's lack of safety awareness, they feared he would accidentally burn the house down or wander off and die of exposure or be hit by a car. They admitted him to the Quality Care facility, and made arrangements for his wife's admission when she is discharged from the hospital. Dr. Zeleski is in a room by himself, in anticipation of his wife's arrival within the next few days. Family members have cautioned the facility that he wandered away from home several times, and stated that they would take legal action if he got outside and was injured. Dr. Zeleski is restless and agitated every evening. His balance is good and he moves quickly. He wears a magnetic wandering bracelet, but has managed to remove it twice. He has left the building and gone outside several times. He usually slips into large groups of visitors who are exiting the building.

Dr. Zeleski often wanders about looking for his wife. He does not remember that she is in the hospital. Sometimes he goes into other residents' rooms and upsets them. He tells you he is going home and argues when reminded that he lives in the facility. He seldom wears a coat or dresses appropriately for the weather. Dr. Zeleski is often so distracted that he does not finish a meal before he is up to wander again. He has lost weight. He has an order for a regular diet with large portions, with nutritional supplements three times daily and PRN. He especially likes the eggnog flavor supplement. You know he also likes tuna salad sandwiches and deviled eggs. He has an order for restraints if he is unmanageable, but these are to be used only as a last resort.

60. Dr. Zeleski is approaching the door when you see him. He says, "Goodbye. I am going home now." What action will you take to keep the resident safe?

_____

_____

_____

_____

_____

61. You are assigned to care for Dr. Zeleski today. Your unit is short of staff, and Dr. Zeleski is very agitated. A number of visitors have been in the facility, and he has tried to slip out several times. Each time staff have retrieved him, but you fear you will be in a resident's room and he will slip out. Should you restrain him to keep him safe? Why or why not? If you elect not to apply restraints, how will you ensure the resident's safety?

_____

_____

_____

_____

62. Dr. Zeleski did not eat his dinner. He got up from the table and started wandering the halls. Almost everyone is in the dining room, and you fear he will slip out the door. When you approach the resident, he says he is "late for work." You walk with him as he heads for the door. How can you assist this resident to eat dinner and keep from leaving the facility?

_____

_____

_____

_____

63. Dr. Zeleski refused to eat his meal. How can you assist in meeting his nutritional needs?

_____

_____

_____

_____

64. Based on the descriptions in your textbook, what type of wanderer is Dr. Zeleski? What does this tell you about his risk for eloping? In addition to the wandering category, does the resident have any other factors that increase his chances of eloping successfully? If so, list them.

_____

_____

_____

_____

65. Why are good teamwork and communication important in the care of this resident?

_____

_____

_____

_____

66. You are asked to attend Dr. Zeleski's care conference. The nurse tells you to think about suggestions to keep the resident safe. What will you suggest?

_____

_____

_____

_____

_____

67. The confused residents in the following figure need attention badly. Identify at least 13 problems in the residents' room.

a. _____

b. _____

c. _____

d. _____

e. _____

f. _____

g. _____

h. _____

i. _____

j. _____

k. _____

l. _____

m. _____

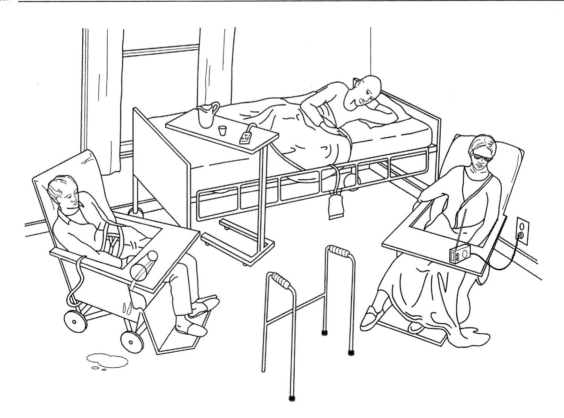

68. Rearrange the letters to form three sentences in the lower grid. (Keep the letters in the same columns; skip a column for a space between words.).

T					E	A		L			E	S		I	E		T	A		S	
T		O	X	O	T	K	K		S	O	E		I	I	C	H		E	T		T	D	S	R	T		N
H	S	A	E	W	P	R	R	E	I	F	N	K	F	F	A	A	L		R	E		R	O	E	I	D	E	S
M	E	T	I	C	H	I	R	T	E	E	I	A	O	V	T	L	E	A	G	E	S	I	E	K	N	A	I	T
E	E	A	M	T	C	A	L	D	B	S	E	R	E	W	I	S	N	T	H	N	T	I	R	E	E	T	E	A

CHAPTER 21

Death and Dying

KEY POINTS

- The nursing assistant is expected to provide care to residents who are dying, and care for the body after death.
- When caring for residents who are dying, the nursing assistant will assist residents and families to meet physical, emotional, psychological, social, and spiritual needs.
- Residents with terminal illness are not expected to recover, but the exact time of death cannot be predicted.
- The nursing assistant's personal beliefs about death and dying will affect the care given to the resident.
- A hospice is an agency that cares for dying residents.
- Hospice care focuses on keeping residents comfortable and allowing them to die with dignity and respect.
- Coping mechanisms are responses to stress and loss that are used to protect self-esteem.
- The five steps in the grieving process are denial, anger, bargaining, depression, and acceptance.
- The resident and family's cultural and religious beliefs about death and dying must be respected.
- Standard precautions are used when caring for the deceased, because the body can be infectious after death.

ACTIVITIES

Vocabulary

Find the words in the puzzle on page 154. In phrases, only the words in italics are hidden in the puzzle. Define each word or phrase.

1. acceptance_____

2. anger_____

3. apathy_____

4. bargaining_____

5. cardiac *arrest* _____

6. code *blue*_____

7. coping *mechanisms* _____

8. denial _____

9. depression _____

10. *DNR* (do not resuscitate) order _____

11. *grieving* process _____

12. hospice _____

13. *rigor* mortis _____

14. shroud _____

15. *terminal* illness _____

b	a	h	o	s	p	i	c	e	f	r	g
E	a	n	d	e	n	i	a	l	i	a	r
s	a	r	g	a	e	O	T	g	c	Q	i
m	p	v	g	e	e	N	o	c	s	t	e
s	a	O	H	a	r	r	e	z	L	s	v
i	t	c	u	P	i	p	E	D	M	e	i
n	h	C	d	D	t	n	v	T	c	r	n
a	y	B	N	a	g	F	i	e	C	r	g
h	C	R	n	T	w	k	p	n	u	a	H
c	w	c	d	u	o	r	h	s	g	l	m
e	e	k	l	a	n	i	m	r	e	t	b
m	A	n	o	i	s	s	e	r	p	e	d

Completion

Fill in the chart to identify the stages of the grieving process and nursing assistant response.

Resident Statement	Stage of Grief	Nursing Assistant Response
16. "I should donate to the cancer charity so they find a cure on time."		
17. "They haven't visited in two days. No one cares about me any more."		
18. "I need to speak with my cousin Charles. We haven't spoken in years, and it's time."		
19. "This diagnosis can't be right. The doctor doesn't know what she's doing."		
20. "This food makes me sick. In fact, I'm sick of all of you. Take this horrible food out of here."		

21. Name the individual who identified and researched the stages of the grieving process.

_____

22. Does each person pass through the stages of the grieving process in order?

_____

23. After moving through a stage of the grieving process into the next stage, does a person ever move backward?

_____

24. Do families or staff ever experience the grieving process?

_____

25. List four ways in which the nursing assistant can assist residents who are having difficulty coping.

_____

_____

_____

_____

26. List at least 10 signs or symptoms of approaching death.

_____

_____

_____

_____

_____

_____

_____

_____

_____

_____

_____

_____

27. Explain why standard precautions must be used when providing postmortem care.

_____

_____

_____

_____

True/False

Mark the following statements true or false.

28. T F The hospice gives postmortem care when the resident is diagnosed with a terminal illness.
29. T F If the resident has a DNR order, CPR must be done if the resident's heart stops beating.
30. T F A terminal illness is a condition from which the resident is expected to recover.
31. T F Death is a natural part of life.
32. T F Some elderly persons see death as a relief from pain and suffering.
33. T F Some people fear death.
34. T F The hospice provides aggressive care for residents who are dying.
35. T F The hospice also provides services to family members.
36. T F Coping mechanisms are used to protect self-esteem.

37. T F   Most people complete the grieving process before death.

38. T F   When a person is dying, vision is the last sensation to be lost.

39. T F   A licensed nurse must provide the care of the body after death.

40. T F   It is not necessary to provide privacy after the resident dies.

41. T F   Rigor mortis is a permanent condition that develops about 10 hours after death.

42. T F   The resident may be incontinent after death.

43. T F   When circulation stops, the blood begins to pool in the lowest areas of the body.

44. T F   Family members should not be left alone with the body after death.

45. T F   When a resident is dying, keep the room dark and very warm.

46. T F   When a resident is dying, you may be unable to hear the blood pressure, yet you can count the respirations.

47. T F   Handling a body roughly can cause permanent marks and bruises.

48. T F   The nursing assistant is not responsible for assisting residents with spiritual needs.

49. T F   The nursing assistant should try to humor the resident who is apathetic.

Developing Greater Insight

Answer the following questions based on this situation.

> Mrs. Kosmacek has a terminal diagnosis, and her condition has been steadily declining. She keeps talking about a trip she plans to take next summer, which is 10 months away. She has been planning this trip and saving her money for many years. She says she is going to Poland to research her ancestry. While she is overseas, she plans to go on to the Vatican to see if she can get a blessing from the pope. She says she is going to make reservations soon and make a large, nonrefundable deposit so she gets the dates and accommodations she wants.

50. How will you react to the resident discussing trip plans?

_____

51. Will you report this conversation to anyone? If so, whom and why?

_____

52. What stage of the grieving process is the resident displaying?

_____

53. Rearrange the letters to form a sentence in the lower grid. (Keep the letters in the same columns; skip a column for a space between words.)

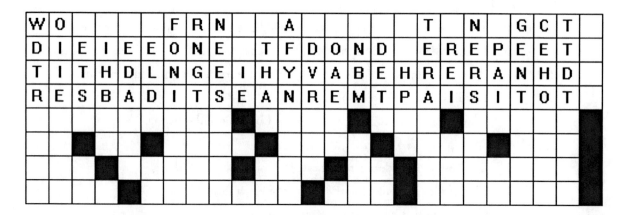

CHAPTER 22

The Nursing Assistant in Home Care

KEY POINTS

- Working in home care provides independence and autonomy to health care workers.

- Most home health care is delivered by home care agencies, which employ an entire interdisciplinary team of home care workers.

- Home health care workers may also visit residents in assisted living facilities.

- The home health care nursing assistant's job description lists your duties and responsibilities. Ask questions and clarify if needed. Make sure you understand what is expected.

- The home health care nursing assistant must learn and respect clients' rights.

- The RN will develop the nursing assistant plan of care, describing duties and care that nursing assistants are expected to provide.

- The home health nursing assistant must plan care around client needs and family routines.

- The home health nursing assistant is responsible for maintaining a comfortable, safe, and sanitary home environment.

- Apply the principles of standard precautions and wash your hands frequently.

- The home health nursing assistant must adapt nursing assistant skills and available supplies to provide nursing care in the home.

- Always be alert to unsafe practices, conditions, or situations.

- The home health nursing assistant is responsible for planning his or her assignment and completing it within a designated period of time.

- Think about your assignment, and plan your work before arriving at the client's home.

- The home health nursing assistant is a guest in the client's home.

- Be pleasant, courteous, and tactful when dealing with the client's family.

- If the client or a family member informs you of new problems with eating, getting into or out of bed, maintaining continence or using the bathroom, bathing, dressing, or safety, notify the supervising nurse.

- Client care records are documentation forms that are used for communication and reimbursement purposes.

- Time and travel records are reports showing how you spent your time.

- For personal safety, be alert to the conditions and people around you.

ACTIVITIES

Vocabulary

Define the following terms in the spaces provided, and answer the questions to show your understanding of these documents.

1. time and travel records _____

2. client care records _____

3. List five things you will document on the time and travel record each day.
   _____
   _____
   _____
   _____
   _____
   _____

4. List two main things you will document on client care records.
   _____
   _____

Completion

Complete the following statements about the role and responsibilities of the home care nursing assistant by selecting the correct term from the list provided here.

adapt	decision making	identification	needs
agencies	flexible	institutional	routines
alert	food guide pyramid	insurance	safe environment
assisted living facilities	glasses	job description	safety
bathroom	guest	kitchen	solve problems
communication	healing	less	supervision
continuity of care			

5. Home care encourages individual _____.

6. When a client receives home care, _____ risks are minimized.

7. Home care promotes _____.

8. Home care is usually _____ expensive than other forms of care.

9. The psychological benefits, comfort, and security of being at home may promote _____.

10. Most home health care is delivered by home care _____.

11. In addition to working in clients' homes, home care workers may also visit persons in _____.

12. The nursing assistant who works in home care must be _____, able to _____, and know when to call for help.

13. The nursing assistant who works in home care must have good _____ skills.

14. The nursing assistant who works in home care must not need intense _____.

15. The duties of the home health nursing assistant are planned around client _____ and family _____.

16. You will need to learn to _____ your nursing assistant skills and available supplies to provide nursing care in the home.

17. The nursing assistant is responsible for maintaining a _____.

18. Client meals and menus should be based on the _____.

19. When washing dishes by hand, wash _____ first.

20. Two areas of the home with great potential for infection are the _____ and _____.

21. The nursing assistant is a _____ in the home of the client and family.

22. Always wear your _____ badge.

23. When working in the community, always be _____ to conditions and people around you.

24. If you are using your personal vehicle to commute to and from work, you should always have _____ on the vehicle.

25. The nursing assistant who works in home care will have a _____ describing the responsibilities of the position.

26. Think _____ at all times.

True/False

Mark the following statements true or false.

27. T   F   The home care nursing assistant must be self-motivated and self-directed.

28. T   F   Plan meals with the client or a family member.

29. T   F   No formal listing of client rights is used for home health care, because clients live in their own homes.

30. T   F   Thaw frozen foods on the countertop.

31. T   F   Contact the physician promptly to report new information.

32. T   F   All home care clients are elderly.

33. T   F   The nursing assistant is responsible for washing the client's clothing and bed linen.

34. T   F   If you work during the night, you may sleep if the client is asleep.

35. T   F   Using home care workers in this manner promotes the "aging in place" philosophy of the assisted living facility.

36. T   F   The RN is responsible for monitoring the clients' home for problems that could cause falls or other injuries.

37. T   F   The nursing assistant should always do what family members want.

38. T   F   The RN will identify your duties and the care you will be expected to provide.

39. T   F   You must only document care given. The RN will document nursing observations.

40. T   F   Store fresh food and leftovers in covered, wrapped containers.

41. T   F   Home care nursing assistants do not assist clients with medications.

42. T   F   Always wash your hands for at least 15 to 20 seconds before handling food.

43. T   F   It is not necessary to use standard precautions when working in home care.

44. T   F   Leftover food should be refrigerated within four hours.

45. T   F   If the client's home needs modifications, an occupational therapist may be asked to make a home visit to make recommendations.

46. T F   Rearrange things if something in the client's home is inconvenient for you.

47. T F   The nursing assistant must do the heavy cleaning at least once each week.

48. T F   The nursing assistant is expected to care for the client's medical equipment, furnishings, and supplies.

49. T F   No special knowledge or preparation is necessary to care for a client in the home.

50. T F   Always take the client's side in family disputes.

Computations

Compute the time spent in each case.

Arrival Time	Departure Time	Time Spent
51. 8:15 a.m.	8:50 a.m.	_____
52. 10:05 a.m.	11:15 a.m.	_____
53. 11:20 a.m.	1:05 p.m.	_____
54. 2:10 p.m.	3:15 p.m.	_____
55. 3:45 p.m.	4:30 p.m.	_____

Short Answer

Write the information in the space provided.

56. List 10 guidelines for avoiding personal liability when providing home care.

_____

_____

_____

_____

_____

_____

_____

_____

_____

_____

57. List at least eight members of the typical home care team.

_____

_____

_____

_____

_____

_____

_____

_____

58. List at least five emergency telephone contacts that you should have available for each client.

_____

_____

_____

_____

_____

59. List the four areas of the home with the greatest risk for injury.

_____

_____

_____

_____

60. List at least four things that you should pack in your nursing bag.

_____

_____

_____

_____

61. List six changes in condition that should be reported to your supervisor for further nursing assessment.

_____

_____

_____

_____

_____

_____

62. List three changes in condition that require immediate reporting to your supervisor.

_____

_____

_____

63. List at least 10 guidelines for maintaining personal safety.

_____

_____

_____

_____

_____

_____

_____

_____

_____

_____

Developing Greater Insight

Answer the following questions based on the situation below.

Mr. Hillhouse has terminal cancer. You will spend an entire shift with him. You must give him a bed bath, change his linen, and prepare his meals. The client enjoys playing cards and dominoes. Your odometer reads 53,726 when you leave your home, and 53,735 when you arrive at the client's home. Your time in is 7:00 a.m. You leave the client's home at 3:40 p.m. Your odometer reads 53,735 when you leave the client's home and 53,744 when you arrive at your own home.

64. Compute the total time spent with the client.

_____

65. Compute the total mileage.

_____

66. Your work is done by 1:00 p.m. and the client is watching television. He says he does not want to take a nap. Mr. Hillhouse says he is bored with the soap operas. Describe your actions.

_____

_____

_____

_____

_____

_____

Mrs. Waggoner is receiving home care services after having a stroke. She has been complaining of arthritis pain. She says she does not take any pain medication because she does not want to become a "drug addict." Today, she is complaining of an intermittent crushing pain in the center of her chest, radiating to her jaw. You take her vital signs and find they are within normal limits.

67. Do you think this pain is related to the client's arthritis pain?

_____

68. What is the the first action you will take?

_____

You are on the telephone waiting to speak with your supervisor, who is on another line. Mrs. Waggoner suddenly becomes short of breath. You notice her lips and nail beds are slightly blue in color.

69. What action will you take?

_____

Mrs. Waggoner's daughter and grandchildren arrive for a visit while the client is having chest pain. The client is so short of breath that she can barely speak and states that she does not want her grandchildren to see her like this.

70. What action will you take?

_____

CHAPTER 23

Employment Opportunities

KEY POINTS

- There are many employment opportunities for nursing assistants.

- Finding employment is a full-time job.

- The best time to look for a job is early in the day.

- It is helpful to list your skills, activities, background, and experience before preparing your resume.

- Your resume should appear as professional as possible, and accurately reflect your education, experience, skills, and interests.

- Information such as race, age, sex, height, weight, national origin, marital and family status, and religion should not be listed on your resume.

- The state employment commission, private employers, government personnel offices, public libraries, newspaper ads, employment agencies, colleges and trade schools, clubs, newsletters, friends, and relatives are all sources of potential job leads.

- Present a professional appearance when you arrive for a job interview.

- Honesty, dependability, and a positive attitude are important characteristics of the nursing assistant.

- This class is just the beginning of your education; you will continue to learn and grow throughout your health care career.

- If resignation is necessary, always give proper notice to the employer.

ACTIVITIES

Vocabulary

Write the words forming the circle and define them in the spaces provided.

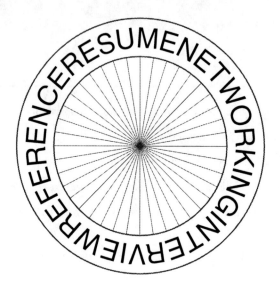

1. _____
2. _____
3. _____
4. _____

Find the words in the puzzle below. In phrases, only the words in italics are hidden in the puzzle. Define each word or phrase.

5. application _____

6. reverse *chronological* order _____

7. *cover* letter _____

8. personal *data* _____

9. *extracurricular* activities _____

10. job *objective* _____

e	y	b	d	v	i	n	n	r	o	q	k	c	c	x
h	x	b	x	s	v	o	r	w	i	a	o	h	l	e
x	d	t	b	l	h	h	p	n	s	v	r	l	j	y
f	t	u	r	x	m	x	q	l	e	o	x	j	m	c
k	t	m	b	a	l	g	q	r	n	a	u	v	y	f
v	d	w	a	n	c	i	z	o	f	u	k	l	j	e
s	v	o	u	q	z	u	l	n	d	m	j	o	x	v
j	s	i	v	p	p	o	r	y	n	u	j	w	j	i
s	d	z	u	v	g	h	d	r	f	f	b	p	v	t
y	o	e	h	i	t	m	z	i	i	o	d	o	r	c
e	e	d	c	p	x	d	q	r	k	c	n	o	i	e
a	p	a	b	g	o	t	l	j	a	u	u	p	k	j
t	l	d	w	j	a	t	z	b	a	t	g	l	p	b
a	q	c	h	f	x	x	t	n	c	c	r	d	a	o
d	v	p	n	o	i	t	a	c	i	l	p	p	a	r

Completion

Complete the following statements by selecting the correct term from the list provided here.

attendance	employment	ink	physical	thank
avoid	eye contact	negative	positive	tuberculosis
continuing education	first impression	on time	positive attitude	weak
criminal history check	follows	permission	prepared	written
drug testing	handshake	personal	responsibilities	
early	identify	photo	shake hands	

11. Be _____ when looking for a job.

12. You will need a _____ identification when applying for a job.

13. Get _____ before listing someone as a reference.

14. Before applying for a job, _____ situations and circumstances that could interfere with your ability to do the job.

15. Your state _____ office has information and resources to assist you in getting a job.

16. Avoid listing _____ information such as race, age, or gender on your resume.

17. Call potential employers _____ in the day.

18. Fill out the application in _____.

19. Your appearance during the interview is very important and helps you make a positive _____.

20. _____ when you are introduced to the interviewer.

21. A _____ handshake may send a negative message.

22. Make good _____ with the interviewer.

23. During the interview, avoid making _____ comments about a former employer.

24. During the interview, _____ discussing your personal life or financial problems.

25. Do not accept a position if you cannot fulfill the _____.

26. Always _____ the employer for the interview.

27. Close the interview with a firm _____.

28. In some states, employers are required to conduct a _____ on each applicant.

29. Many employers require a _____ examination and _____ before hiring an applicant.

30. The employer will probably perform two-step _____ testing on each new employee.

31. Arrive for work _____, in proper uniform, and be prepared to work.

32. Maintain a _____ and be willing to learn new things.

33. Good _____ is very important.

34. Your work record _____ you.

35. You should give _____ notice of resignation.

36. The federal rules require nursing assistants to complete at least 12 hours of _____ each year.

37. Always leave your job on a _____ note.

True/False

Mark the following statements true or false.

38. T　F　At the job interview, you should wait to be invited before sitting.

39. T　F　Body language is not important during the interview.

40. T　F　When filling out an application, write "see resume," and attach your resume.

41. T　F　Your interests and volunteer activities may have helped you develop skills and talents that are useful on the job.

42. T　F　Your resume may be handwritten.

43. T　F　Print your resume on newsprint-quality paper.

44. T　F　Send an individualized cover letter each time you mail a resume.

45. T　F　Do not list employers outside the health care field on your resume.

46. T　F　The job history section of your resume should be written in chronological order.

47. T　F　There is no cost for state employment commission services.

48. T　F　During the job interview, avoid discussing negative traits unless you are specifically asked to do so.

49. T　F　Ask questions about the salary and benefits early in the interview.

50. T　F　Make sure you inform the interviewer of your demands for time off.

51. T　F　Call the facility well in advance if you must be absent from work.

52. T　F　Staff and residents depend on you to be at work on time, when scheduled.

53. T　F　The nursing assistant class is the beginning of your education; you will continue to learn and grow throughout your health care career.

54. T　F　Honesty, dependability, and a positive attitude are important characteristics.

55. T　F　It is not necessary to give notice of resignation if you have another job offer that pays more.

Completion

56. Complete the employment application.

BRIDGEWATER SKILLED CARE FACILITY
Application for Employment

1. Full Name   Miss
                 Mrs.
                 Mr.   _____
                        Last   First   Middle   Maiden

                        _____
                        Street and Number or Rural Route

                        _____
                        City, State and ZIP Code

                        _____
                        County   Telephone or nearest - Specify

                        Social Security Number _____

2. Birth Date _____ Age _____ Birthplace _____

3. Physical Data: Height _____ Weight _____

4. Family and Marital Status: Single ____ Married ____ Widowed ____ Separated ____ Divorced ____
    Husband or Wife's Name _____
    Are you self-supporting? _____ Number of children and ages _____
    Other dependents (specify) _____

5. Person to notify in case of emergency:
    Name _____   Name of parents _____
    Address _____   Address _____
    _____   _____
    Telephone _____   Telephone _____
    Relationship _____

6. Education: List in this order --- High School, College. You must give complete addresses. Also please note if you did not graduate from high school whether or not you have a GED certificate.

School	Address	City	State	Year

7. Work or Vocational Experience: Give most recent first.

Name of Institution or Company	Complete Address	Type of Work	Dates

8. Have you ever been arrested for anything other than minor traffic violations? Yes ____ No ____
    If yes, explain.

9. Are you now or have you been addicted to the use of alcohol or habit-forming drugs: Yes ____ No ____
    If yes, explain.

10. References: Name three people who know your qualifications or who know your character. They must not be related to you.
    Name _____
    Address _____
    Name _____
    Address _____
    Name _____
    Address _____

11. What are your reasons for wishing to work at this facility? Please answer this question in paragraph form on the back of this application.

57. Practice writing a resignation letter in the space provided.

_____
Date

Dear _____

Please accept this letter as my written notice of resignation from my position as

_____. My resignation is effective as of _____.

Working here at _____ has given me an opportunity

to _____.

I find I must leave because _____.

Thank you for giving me this opportunity to learn and grow.

Sincerely,

_____

Developing Greater Insight

Answer the questions based on your knowledge of factors that affect communication. If necessary, review the communication information in Chapter 6 of your textbook.

58. The poem _Messengers_ on page 41 of your workbook notes that the eyes are the messengers of the soul. How can you use your eyes to your best advantage in communicating during the job interview?

_____

_____

_____

_____

59. How can you use your body language to your best advantage during the job interview?

_____

_____

_____

_____

60. Rearrange the letters to form a sentence in the lower grid. (Keep the letters in the same columns; skip a column for a space between words.)

H			R	U		A		R			M	S	I	A			N		
Y	O	A	N	S		T		E	G	I	A	T	C	V	E	T	F	N	T
C	H	U	D	E	C	A	E	P	E	P	E	I	D	S	S	O	A	T	T
I	E	N	E	A	R	S	R	D	I	S	I	P	O	I	B	A	A	I	T
H	T	A	N	D	T	Y	I	N	O	S	T	N	S	R	T	I	L	T	T
							■												
	■				■		■								■				
					■				■										■
												■		■					
		■							■										

CHAPTER 24

Surviving a Survey

KEY POINTS

- Long-term care facilities must meet quality standards to operate.

- Licensure is a process in which the facility is inspected for a state license to operate.

- Certification is necessary if long-term care facilities accept Medicare and Medicaid money as reimbursement for resident care.

- Accreditation is a voluntary process in which facilities are inspected to ensure that they meet high quality standards of resident care.

- OSHA inspects long-term care facilities to monitor infection control and safety practices that affect employees.

- Many agencies survey health care facilities, so the facility must be survey-ready every day.

- Most surveys are unannounced.

- Long-term care facility surveyors usually observe the nursing assistant giving direct resident care.

- Infection control practices are a very important part of all surveys.

- The nursing assistant is responsible for learning and following the policies and procedures of the long-term care facility.

- Following facility policies and doing things the way you were taught will prevent problems during surveys.

- The nursing assistant is responsible for providing care that complies with accepted standards of practice for health care providers.

ACTIVITIES

Vocabulary

1. Complete the crossword puzzle by using the hints and definitions listed.

Across

1 Occupational Safety and Health Administration

3 Joint Commission on Accreditation for Healthcare Organizations

4 representatives of a private or governmental agency who review long-term care facility policies, procedures, and practices for quality of care

6 The _____ conference is a meeting between surveyors and facility administration upon completion of a survey to discuss the surveyors' findings and the nature of deficiencies.

10 an inspection process for facilities that accept state or federal funds as payment for health care

12 a state permit allowing the long-term care facility to operate

14 a review and evaluation to ensure that long-term care facilities are maintaining acceptable standards of practice, quality of care, and quality of life for residents

15 An _____ survey lasts longer than originally anticipated, so surveyors can examine resident care and facility practices in greater detail.

Down

2 process that health care facilities participate in voluntarily to ensure that high standards of care are maintained

5 The _____ conference is a meeting between surveyors and facility administration to discuss the purpose of a survey; it is always conducted at the beginning of a survey.

7 Quality _____ is an internal review made by facility staff to identify problems and find solutions for improvement.

8 a written notice of inadequate care or a substandard practice

9 written notice that informs the health care agency of alleged violations; some agencies also inform the facility of the time frame in which the condition must be corrected

11 The plan of _____ is a written plan submitted by the health care agency in response to deficient survey findings; it lists what corrections will be made, by whom, who will monitor the changes, and what will be done to prevent similar deficiencies in the future.

13 Centers for Medicare and Medicaid Services

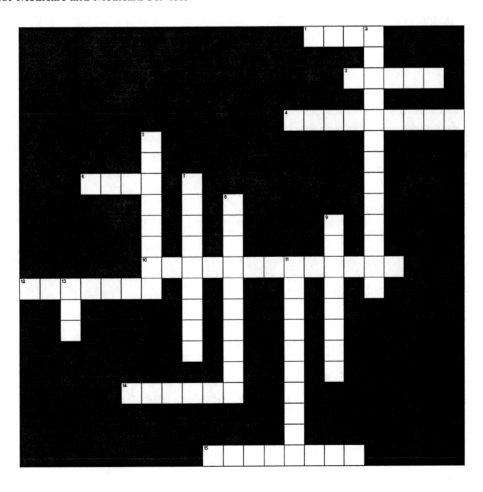

Completion

Complete the chart to indicate which activities are the nursing assistant's responsibility during a survey.

Activity	Nursing Assistant Responsibility	
	Yes	No
2. Wash your hands before and after care of each resident.		
3. Give each resident a complete bath or shower.		
4. Dress each resident in his or best clothes.		
5. Tell surveyors everything they need to know.		
6. Respect resident rights.		
7. Serve meals promptly.		
8. Make sure residents' faces, hands, and clothing are clean after meals.		
9. Avoid the surveyors who are in the facility to see nurses and residents.		
10. Ask residents to behave while surveyors are in the facility.		
11. Answer call signals promptly.		
12. Release restraints every three hours.		
13. Leave restraints off when surveyors are in the facility.		
14. Follow facility policies and procedures.		
15. Know the facility fire and safety codes, and explain them if asked.		
16. If a surveyor watches you doing resident care, inform the resident that you are being tested.		
17. Remove residents' personal items that collect dust until surveyors leave the building.		
18. Give the care listed on the care plan and know the residents' goals.		
19. Document your care and ADLs in advance.		
20. Smile and speak to surveyors if you pass them in the hallway.		
21. Wear gloves for all resident contact.		
22. Make the beds as soon as surveyors arrive.		
23. Explain procedures to residents before beginning them.		
24. Tend to the needs of incontinent residents promptly.		
25. Avoid showing surveyors the peri-care procedure.		
26. Record intake and output for all of your assigned residents.		
27. Communicate with confused residents when giving care.		
28. Make sure all residents have the call signal within reach.		
29. Inform surveyors of all the facilities' problems.		
30. Close the door and privacy curtain when you are giving care.		

Matching

Match the terms and description.

Description

31. _____ emphasizes maintaining a homelike environment

32. _____ federal agency that is the primary regulatory body for nursing homes

33. _____ agency responsible for employee safety

34. _____ nursing home inspectors who arrive at facility unannounced

35. _____ clean linen carts and soiled hampers placed at least one room apart

36. _____ composed of facility employees; identifies and corrects problems and maintains quality

37. _____ based on MDS and designed to maintain or improve residents

38. _____ primary accrediting agency

39. _____ a major focus of state and federal surveys

40. _____ may be assessed for deficiencies and negative resident outcomes

41. _____ inform the nurse promptly

42. _____ examines conditions in great detail to determine if a danger to residents exists

Terms

a. Quality Assurance Committee
b. JCAHO
c. extended survey
d. care plan
e. monetary penalties
f. IV pump alarm sounds
g. meal service
h. OSHA
i. surveyors
j. CMS
k. OBRA nursing home rules
l. infection control in hallways

Completion

Complete the following statements by selecting the correct term from the list provided here.

accommodate	contamination	identity	normal
advance	continuing education classes	important	observations
anticipate	control	infection control	post
care plans	correcting	interview	resident rights
clean	deficiencies	introduce	sign
complaints	guests	licensure	temperature

43. It is illegal to notify the facility of a survey in _____.

44. Surveyors want to see resident care and facility routines on a _____ day.

45. Long-term care facilities have regular _____ surveys every 9 to 15 months.

46. Surveyors visit facilities in response to _____ from residents and families.

47. During the initial tour of the facility, surveyors will make _____ of residents and facility conditions.

48. Surveyors are responsible for identifying _____.

49. Facilities are responsible for _____ the problems identified by surveyors.

50. Surveyors do not disclose the _____ of individuals who call the hotline about the facility.

51. The surveyors' first round is very _____ to the survey process.

52. During the survey, a _____ is posted on the door to notify everyone that a survey is in process.

53. Surveyors will _____ alert residents and conduct a resident council meeting.

54. Maintaining proper food _____ is very important.

55. Surveyors verify that staff have completed the required _____ each year.

56. Surveyors also evaluate how well staff protects _____.

57. The facility is required to _____ resident needs as much as possible.

58. Surveyors are _____ in the facility.

59. If a surveyor watches you giving care, you should _____ the surveyor to the resident.

60. Surveyors review resident _____ in advance, so they have an idea of the care that should be given.

61. Remember that _____ is a major area of deficiencies.

62. Avoid _____ of environmental surfaces with your used gloves.

63. Always try to _____ and prevent problems.

64. Give residents as much _____ over daily routines as possible.

65. Facilities must _____ the written survey report.

66. Make sure your assigned residents are _____ and odor-free.

Developing Greater Insight

Answer the following questions based on this situation.

> Surveyors arrive at the facility at 8:15 p.m. Sunday evening. The staff on duty are startled at the time and day of their arrival. The nurse has called the administrator and director of nursing at home, and they will be coming into the facility. In the meantime, the surveyor is making rounds with the RN supervisor. You estimate that they will be in your section in about 15 minutes. You have given one shower. You cannot remember if you removed the soiled towels from the shower room. You still have one shower to give and have put several residents to bed. Mr. Bazeley is in bed, but throws his covers off frequently. Tyrone suggested that you tuck the sheets in tightly all the way around the bed so he cannot expose himself, but you have not done this yet. Miss Tichelbaut is also in bed, but she has been yelling. As you walk down the hallway, you smell something unpleasant. You look to the right and notice that Mrs. Abebe has been incontinent of stool on the floor of her room, and she needs to be cleaned up. At this point, you are feeling stressed and overwhelmed. You take several deep breaths and determine to do well on this survey.

67. What action will you take first?

_____

_____

_____

_____

68. What will you do next?

_____

_____

_____

_____

69. Should you tuck the sheets in tightly to prevent Mr. Bazeley from exposing himself? Why or why not? What can the nursing assistant do to keep him from exposing himself?

---

70. Will Miss Tichelbaut's yelling negatively affect the survey? What can the nursing assistant do about the yelling?

---

71. Rearrange the letters to form a sentence in the lower grid. (Keep the letters in the same columns; skip a column for a space between words.)

	H	A		T		B	I		R			S	A	Y
I	R	E		T	O		E	E	E	L	U		S	T	R
S	T	E	A	N	U	R	S	V	N	S	Y	A	V	S	I
T	V	E	N	D	Y	S	H	O	U	G	D	R	D	E	Y
			■							■					
				■							■				
			■		■			■							
■						■					■				

PART II

Beginning Procedure Actions

Procedure Completion Actions

Student Performance Record

BEGINNING PROCEDURE ACTIONS

Beginning Procedure Action	Rationale
1. Assemble equipment and take it to the resident's room.	Improves efficiency of the procedure. Ensures you do not have to leave the room.
2. Knock on the resident's door and identify yourself by name and title.	Respects the resident's right to privacy. Notifies the resident who is giving care.
3. Identify the resident by checking the identification bracelet, or other method according to facility policy.	Ensures that you are caring for the correct resident.
4. Ask visitors to leave the room and advise them where they may wait.	Respects the resident's right to privacy. Advising visitors where to wait demonstrates hospitality.
5. Explain what you are going to do and how the resident can assist. Answer questions about the procedure.	Informs the resident of what is going to be done and what to expect. Gives the resident an opportunity to get information about the procedure and the extent of resident participation.
6. Provide privacy by closing the door, privacy curtain, and window curtains.	Respects the resident's right to privacy. All three should be closed even if the resident is alone in the room.
7. Wash your hands or use an alcohol-based hand cleaner.	Applies the principles of standard precautions. Prevents the spread of microorganisms.
8. Set up the necessary equipment at the bedside. Open trays and packages. Position items within easy reach. Avoid positioning a container for soiled items in a manner that requires crossing over clean items to access it.	Prepares for the procedure. Ensures that the equipment and supplies are conveniently positioned and readily available. Reduces the risk of cross-contamination.
9. Position the resident for the procedure. Ask an assistant to help, if necessary, or support the resident with pillows and props. Make sure the resident is comfortable and can maintain the position throughout the procedure. Drape the resident for modesty, even if you and the resident are alone in the room.	Ensures that the resident is in the correct position for the procedure. Ensures that the resident is supported and can maintain the position without discomfort. Respects the resident's modesty and dignity.
10. Raise the bed to a comfortable working height.	Prevents back strain and injury caused by bending at the waist.
11. Apply gloves if contact with blood, moist body fluids (except sweat), mucous membranes, secretions, excretions, or nonintact skin is likely.	Applies the principles of standard precautions. Protects the nursing assistant and the resident from transmission of pathogens.

12. Apply a gown if your uniform will have substantial contact with linen or other articles contaminated with blood, moist body fluids (except sweat), secretions, or excretions.

Applies the principles of standard precautions. Protects your uniform from contamination with bloodborne pathogens.

13. Apply a gown, mask, and eye protection if splashing of blood or moist body fluids is likely.

Applies the principles of standard precautions. Protects the nursing assistant's mucous membranes, uniform, and skin from accidental splashing of bloodborne pathogens.

14. Lower the side rail on the side where you are working. (Raise the rail if you must leave the bedside temporarily.)

Provides an obstacle free area in which to work.

PROCEDURE COMPLETION ACTIONS

Procedure Completion Action	Rationale
1. Remove gloves.	Prevents contamination of environmental surfaces from the gloves.
2. Check to make sure the resident is comfortable and in good alignment.	All body systems function better when the body is correctly aligned. The resident is more comfortable when the body is in good alignment.
3. Replace the bed covers, then remove any drapes used.	Provides warmth and security.
4. Elevate the side rails, if used, before leaving the bedside.	Prevents contamination of the side rails from gloves. Promotes resident's right to a safe environment. Prevents accidents and injuries.
5. Remove other personal protective equipment, if worn, and discard according to facility policy.	Prevents unnecessary environmental contamination from used gloves and protective equipment.
6. Wash your hands or use an alcohol-based hand cleaner.	Applies the principles of standard precautions. Prevents the spread of microorganisms.
7. Return the bed to the lowest horizontal position.	Promotes resident's right to a safe environment. Prevents accidents and injuries.
8. Open the privacy and window curtains.	Privacy is no longer necessary unless preferred by the resident.
9. Leave the resident in a safe and comfortable position, with the call signal and needed personal items within reach.	Prevents accidents and injuries. Ensures that help is available. Eliminates the need to call or stretch for needed personal items.
10. Wash your hands or use an alcohol-based hand cleaner.	Although the hands were washed previously, they have contacted the resident and other items in the room. Wash them again before leaving to prevent potential transfer of microorganisms to areas outside the resident's unit.
11. Inform visitors that they may return to the room.	Demonstrates courtesy to visitors and resident.

12. Report completion of the procedure and any abnormalities or other observations.	Informs the supervisor that your assigned task has been completed, so further care can be planned and you can be reassigned to other duties. Notifies the licensed nurse of abnormalities and changes in the resident's condition that require further assessment.
13. Document the procedure and your observations.	Ongoing progress and care given is documented. Provides a legal record. Informs other members of the interdisciplinary team of the care given.

STUDENT PERFORMANCE RECORD

Feel free to duplicate the following forms. Retain copies in your class file, as appropriate.

STUDENT PERFORMANCE RECORD

Nursing Assistant Name (Last, First)   **Social Security Number**

(Program Name, Location)

Dates of Class ___/___/___ to ___/___/___   S = **Satisfactory Performance**
                    mm dd yyyy   mm dd yyyy   U = **Unsatisfactory Performance**

                                                          ★ = **See comments**

☆ **Program Code Number** ☆   Ints. = **Initials**

                                                         N/A = **Not Applicable**

Place a full signature here to correspond with each set of initials on the form.

Initials	Corresponding Signature of Instructor	Title

No.	PROCEDURAL GUIDELINES	CLASSROOM			SKILLS LAB			CLINICAL		
		S/U	Date	Ints.	S/U	Date	Ints.	S/U	Date	Ints.
SECTION I										
1. Handwashing										
2. Applying and Removing Personal Protective Equipment										
3. Emergency Care for the Resident Who Has Fainted										
4. Emergency Care for the Resident Who Is Having a Seizure										
5. Emergency Care for Falls and Suspected Fractures										
6. Application of Cold Packs to Strains and Bruises										
7. Emergency Care for a Resident with Burns										
8. Emergency Care for Controlling Bleeding										
9. Emergency Care for Vomiting and Aspiration										
10. Emergency Care for Clearing the Obstructed Airway in a Conscious Adult Who Is Sitting or Standing										
11. Emergency Care for Clearing the Obstructed Airway in an Unconscious Adult										

No. PROCEDURAL GUIDELINES	CLASSROOM			SKILLS LAB			CLINICAL		
	S/U	Date	Ints.	S/U	Date	Ints.	S/U	Date	Ints.
SECTION II PERSONAL CARE SKILLS									
12. Moving the Resident to the Side of the Bed									
13. Turning the Resident on the Side Toward You									
14. Turning the Resident on the Side Toward You with a Lift (Draw) Sheet									
15. Turning the Resident on the Side Away from You									
16. Assisting the Resident to Move to the Head of the Bed									
17. Moving the Resident to the Head of the Bed with a Lifting (Draw) Sheet									
18. Moving the Resident Up in Bed with One Assistant									
19. Assisting the Resident to Sit Up on the Side of the Bed									
20. Assisting the Resident to Transfer to Chair or Wheelchair, One Person, with Transfer Belt									
21. Assisting the Resident to Transfer to Chair or Wheelchair, Two Persons, with Transfer Belt									
22. Assisting the Resident to Transfer from Bed to Chair or Wheelchair, One Assistant									
23. Transferring the Resident Using a Mechanical Lift									
24. Sliding Board Transfer from Bed to Wheelchair									
25. Transferring the Resident from Wheelchair to Toilet									
26. Transferring the Resident from Bed to Stretcher									
27. Positioning the Resident in a Chair or Wheelchair									
28. Assisting with Wheelchair Pushups									
29. Leaning to the Side for Pressure Relief									
30. Ambulating the Resident with a Gait Belt									
31. Making the Unoccupied Bed									
32. Making the Occupied Bed									

STUDENT PERFORMANCE RECORD *(continued)*

No.	PROCEDURAL GUIDELINES	CLASSROOM			SKILLS LAB			CLINICAL		
		S/U	Date	Ints.	S/U	Date	Ints.	S/U	Date	Ints.
33.	Changing the Resident's Gown									
34.	Brushing and Flossing the Resident's Teeth									
35.	Special Oral Hygiene									
36.	Denture Care									
37.	Giving a Bed Bath									
38.	Giving a Partial Bath									
39.	Waterless Bed Bath									
40.	Assisting the Resident with a Tub or Shower Bath									
41.	Female Perineal Care									
42.	Male Perineal Care									
43.	Giving a Back Rub									
44.	Shampooing the Hair									
45.	Combing the Hair									
46.	Shaving the Male Resident									
47.	Hand and Fingernail Care									
48.	Foot and Toenail Care									
49.	Applying Antiembolism Stockings									
50.	Assisting the Resident with Dressing									
51.	Feeding the Dependent Resident									
52.	Assisting the Resident with a Bedpan									
53.	Assisting the Male Resident with a Urinal									
54.	Providing Indwelling Catheter Care									
55.	Emptying the Urinary Drainage Bag									
56.	Measuring Urinary Output									
57.	Collecting a Routine Urine Specimen									
58.	Collecting the Midstream (Clean-Catch) Urine Specimen									
59.	Administering a Cleansing Enema									
60.	Administering a Commercially Prepared Enema									
61.	Collecting a Stool Specimen									
62.	Applying a Vest Restraint									
63.	Applying a Belt Restraint									
64.	Applying an Extremity Restraint									

Page 3 of 5

No. PROCEDURAL GUIDELINES	CLASSROOM			SKILLS LAB			CLINICAL		
	S/U	Date	Ints.	S/U	Date	Ints.	S/U	Date	Ints.
65. Measuring an Oral Temperature with a Glass Thermometer									
66. Measuring an Oral Temperature with an Electronic Thermometer									
67. Measuring a Rectal Temperature with a Glass Thermometer									
68. Measuring a Rectal Temperature with an Electronic Thermometer									
69. Measuring an Axillary Temperature with a Glass Thermometer									
70. Measuring an Axillary Temperature with an Electronic Thermometer									
71. Measuring a Tympanic Temperature									
72. Taking the Radial Pulse									
73. Counting Respirations									
74. Using the Stethoscope									
75. Measuring the Blood Pressure									
76. Measuring Weight and Height									
77. Admitting the Resident									
78. Transferring the Resident									
79. Discharging the Resident									
80. Passive Range-of-Motion Exercises									
81. Making a Trochanter Roll									
82. Taking Blood Pressure with an Electronic Blood Pressure Apparatus									
83. Using a Pulse Oximeter									
84. Opening a Sterile Package									
85. Applying Sterile Gloves									
86. Postmortem Care									
Appendix Procedures									
Head-Tilt, Chin-Lift Maneuver									
Jaw-Thrust Maneuver									
Mouth-to-Mask Ventilation									
Adult CPR, One Rescuer									
Adult CPR, Two Rescuers									
Positioning the Resident in the Recovery Position									
Procedure for Cardiac Emergencies and Use of an Elevator									
Measuring Blood Pressure (One-Step Procedure)									
Alternate Methods of Documenting Meal Intake									

STUDENT PERFORMANCE RECORD *(continued)*

No.	PROCEDURAL GUIDELINES	CLASSROOM			SKILLS LAB			CLINICAL		
		S/U	Date	Ints.	S/U	Date	Ints.	S/U	Date	Ints.
List State-Specific Procedures Below										

Comments (Include date and signature/initials)

Feel free to duplicate the performance record. Fill in the skills the student has completed. Retain the original in the master class file.

PART III

Nursing Assistant Written Test Overview

STANDARDIZED TESTING

The state certification test you will be taking is a *standardized test*. This means it was written in such a way that it will be fair to everyone who takes the test. A test becomes standardized only after having been piloted, used, revised, and used again until it shows consistent results. The purpose of a standardized test is to establish an average score, or norm. This allows the results of one person's scores to be compared with the scores of many others across the state or country. A standardized test must be given in the same way each time. This is done by using the same plan and the same directions. The examiner is allowed to give only certain kinds of help. The conditions at all test sites should be similar, and each answer is scored according to definite rules.

The written state test is designed to ensure that you have the knowledge necessary to function safely as an entry-level (beginning) nursing assistant. The test varies by state. For most states, the test has between 50 and 120 questions. You will be given approximately two to four hours to complete the written test, depending on length. Some states include approximately 10 extra questions that are not scored. These are in the process of being standardized for use in future tests. You do not know which questions are scored and which are the unscored questions. The time allowed for completing the test is fairly generous. The test examiner will call "time" near the end of the test to warn you that the end of the allotted time is near.

The written test questions are all in multiple-choice format. Although some questions are difficult, there are no trick questions. Questions are developed by experienced nursing assistant educators and are designed to measure the competency of an average learner. They are not designed to weed out slow learners or reward faster learners. Various terms may be used to describe the person giving care. For testing purposes, the term *nurse aide* is commonly used to describe the caregiver, but other terms, such as *nurse assistant* and *nursing assistant*, may be used in your state. The word *client* is commonly used to describe the individual receiving care, but the terms *patient* and *resident* may also be used. Your examiner will inform you of the proper terms for these individuals. The questions on the test will be placed randomly and will not be grouped together in a specific category or subject.

Many states have a practice test and candidate handbook available. Ask your instructor if these tools are available in your state. They will be invaluable in preparing for your state test. Many of the practice state tests are online at the following testing services:

http://www.capstarlearning.com/nurseaide/
http://www.chauncey.com/
http://www.experioronline.com/
http://www.promissor.com/

Some state nursing assistant registries also maintain Web sites. If your state registry is online, you may wish to check its Web site for information about the state test.

STATE TEST CONTENT

The National Nurse Aide Assessment Program (NNAAP) forms the basis for the examination questions. The purpose of the NNAAP Written (or Oral) Examination is to make sure that you understand the responsibilities and can safely perform the job duties of an entry-level nursing assistant. OBRA '87 was designed to improve the quality of care in long-term care facilities and to define education and examination standards for nursing assistants. Each state is responsible for following the terms of this federal law. The examination is a measure of nursing assistant-related knowledge, skills, and abilities. There are two parts to the examination, written and skills. Both parts are usually given on the same day.

The nursing assistant written test covers the main content areas that you studied in class. These are:

- Physical Care Skills
  - Activities of daily living (ADLs)/Promotion of health and safety
    - hygiene
    - dressing and grooming
    - nutrition and hydration
    - elimination
    - comfort, rest, and sleep
- Basic Nursing Skills
  - Infection control
  - Safety and emergency procedures
  - Therapeutic and technical procedures such as bedmaking, collecting specimens, measuring height and weight, and using restraints
  - Observation, reporting, and data collection
- Restorative Nursing Care Skills/Promotion of Function and Health
  - Preventive health care, such as contracture and pressure ulcer prevention
  - Promotion of client self-care and independence
- Psychosocial Care Skills/Specialized Care
  - Emotional and mental health needs
    - behavior management
    - needs of the dying client
    - sexuality needs
    - cultural and spiritual needs
- Role and Responsibilities of the Nursing Assistant
  - Communication
    - verbal communication
    - nonverbal communication
    - listening
    - clients with special communication problems
  - Resident rights
  - Legal and ethical behavior
  - Responsibilities as a member of the health care team
  - Knowledge of medical terminology and abbreviations

TAKING A MULTIPLE-CHOICE TEST

Most standardized tests use multiple-choice items. This is because multiple-choice questions can measure a variety of learning outcomes, from simple to complex. They also provide the most consistent results. The multiple-choice item consists of a *stem*, which presents a problem situation, and four possible choices, called *alternatives*. The alternatives include the correct answer and several wrong answers called *distractors*. The stem may be a question or incomplete statement, as shown:

- Question form:

  Q. Which of the following people is responsible for taking care of a client?

    a. janitor
    b. administrator
    c. nursing assistant
    d. social worker

■ Incomplete statement form:

Q. The care of a client is the responsibility of a

    a. janitor.
    b. administrator.
    c. nursing assistant.
    d. social worker.

Although worded differently, both stems present the same problem. The alternatives in the examples contain only one correct answer. All distractors are clearly incorrect.

Another type of multiple-choice item is the best-answer format. In this form, the alternatives *may be partially correct*, but one is clearly better than the others. Look at the following example:

■ Best answer form:

Q. Which of the following ethical behaviors is the MOST important?

    a. Maintain a positive attitude.
    b. Act as a responsible employee.
    c. Be courteous to visitors.
    d. Promote quality of life for each client.

Other variations of the best-answer form may ask you what is "the first thing to do," the "most helpful action," the "best response or best answer," or a similar kind of question. Whether the correct-answer or best-answer form is used depends on the information given.

Each multiple-choice question lists four answers. The chance of guessing correctly is only one in four, or 25%. Each test question has only one correct answer. Do not mark more than one answer per item, or the item will be marked wrong. Do not leave answers blank.

STUDY SKILLS

No matter what type of test you take, you must first master the material. Using index cards is an excellent way to do this. The *Nurse Aide Exam Review Cards CD Package* (Delmar, Cengage Learning © 2002) is available in both English and Spanish, and is a perfect companion to your textbook. The *Nurse Aide Exam Review Cards CD Package* was designed to help ensure your success on the state test. This set of 270 flash cards will help you prepare for the state nursing assistant certification exam. Each card contains a sample question on the front and lists the question category, answer, and answer rationale on the back. Conveniently sized and completely portable, these cards are ideal for individual or group study. The cards feature questions corresponding to the National Nurse Aide Assessment Program content outline, study tips, test day hints, and rationales with each answer. They are available as a soft-cover book, with perforated and quartered pages so the study cards can be easily removed. You may wish to prepare additional cards listing vocabulary terms, abbreviations, or questions from your workbook or text. Using index cards to create study or flash cards enables you to test your ability to recognize and retrieve important information.

To study, look at the front of the card and try to answer the question. Turn the card over to see if you are correct. After going through all the cards once, you may wish to shuffle them and review them again. Make sure you know the information and can answer questions in any order.

As you review the cards, begin to sort them into two piles. One pile will be those you know well and the other pile will be those you are having trouble remembering. Once you have two piles, try to learn the most difficult information. Continue reviewing the cards until you have mastered the material. Review the cards several times a day during the time before the exam.

There are a number of advantages to using the card system. First, sorting the cards and preparing extra cards is a good learning experience. Second, the cards are easy and convenient to carry with you in a purse or pocket. You can study them during spare moments throughout the day. Another advantage is that you can use the cards with a friend to quiz each other.

Other Helpful Study Skills

1. Block out a specific time for study. Study your biorhythms to know the time of day when you are functioning at your peak level of performance.

2. Get plenty of sleep.

3. Begin studying well in advance of the state certification test. Schedule your study sessions so you can take a break in between. For example, studying for an hour in the morning and an hour in the evening is more effective than studying for two consecutive hours. Trying to study when you are mentally or physically tired is a waste of time.

4. Study the most difficult material when you are most alert.

5. Control your environment. Do whatever it takes to find a quiet place to study. Get up early in the morning, when everyone else is asleep, or find a quiet corner of the library.

6. Become part of a small, dedicated study group of three to five people, or find a study partner.

7. Eat right, especially protein and complex carbohydrates.

8. Study key concepts by asking yourself, "What are four different ways this concept could be tested?"

9. Learn the rationale behind each issue. Write a brief statement of rationale on the back of each index card with the answer. This has been done for you on the *Nurse Aide Exam Review Cards*. Study all of the information included in the rationale on your study cards. Ask yourself how the information could be tested. Make sure you can apply the principles and rationale to similar situations.

10. You may also create study checklists. Identify all the material for which you are accountable. Break it down into manageable-size lists of steps, notes, and procedures for each item. For example, write down the steps involved for a nursing procedure. Create a separate column for supplies needed and any special information you need to know.

11. Record your notes or study questions on tape. You may play the tape at home or in the car when you are commuting. The CD that accompanies the *Nurse Aide Exam Review Cards* may also be copied on cassette tape for use when you travel.

12. Many excellent tools and resources for studying are available online at http://www.studygs.net.

Stress and Test Anxiety

You may be surprised to learn that stress is normal. A certain amount of stress can be good. Almost everyone has some test anxiety. Studies have shown that mild stress actually improves performance in athletes, entertainers, public speakers, and test takers! Butterflies in the stomach, breathing faster, sweating, and other symptoms are automatic body responses to stressful situations. Stress can sharpen your attention, keep you alert, and give you greater energy. Remember, it is not the stress that is harmful, but your reaction to it. Learn and practice how to control stress. Some stress cannot be avoided, but the date of this exam is known in advance. Try to avoid stressful situations immediately before the test. Prepare yourself physically and mentally.

If you feel stressed immediately before or during the exam, try a deep breathing activity recommended by stress management experts. Breathe slowly and deeply from the diaphragm. Do not move the chest and shoulders. You should feel your abdominal muscles expand when you inhale and relax when you exhale. As you breathe out, your diaphragm and rib muscles seem to relax and your body may seem to sink down into the chair. This helps promote relaxation. Sixty seconds of controlled deep breathing helps relieve stress.

Factors that increase stress and test anxiety are negative thoughts and self-doubt. Perhaps you have thought, "I am going to fail this exam. What will my family or coworkers think if I do not pass?" You must control your reaction to this stress and stop thinking these thoughts. Instead, say to yourself, "I have done this job successfully. I know this material, and did well in class. I am going to pass this examination." View the exam as an opportunity to show what you know and can do. Positive thinking comes before positive action and positive results. Make a conscious effort to stop negative thoughts and force them out by using positive ones.

TAKING THE TEST

To do well on a test, you should be at your best when you start. Eat a good breakfast or lunch. Try to avoid anything that will cause stress. Dress appropriately, according to exam center requirements. Candidates who are not properly attired may be denied admission.

You must be on time to take the state test. If you are late, you may not be admitted. If you miss the test, your testing fees may not be refundable, and you will lose your money. If weather conditions are unsafe, the test may be canceled and rescheduled. If you are absent for a valid emergency, you must submit proof of this emergency to the testing service promptly (usually within 30 days.) Examples of acceptable excuses are a death in the immediate family, disabling traffic accident, illness of yourself or an immediate family member, jury duty, court appearance, or military duty. A service fee may be charged if you miss the test, even if you have proof of an acceptable excuse.

Leave for the test site early enough to arrive on time. Allow a little extra time for minor delays. In some states, you may be required to arrive up to 30 minutes early to allow time for registration, processing, identification verification, and sign-in.

Take a watch and two or three #2, sharpened black lead pencils with erasers. If your state issues an admission letter, bring it with you and present it to the examiner. Most states have a list of supplies or identification that you must bring to be admitted to the test. Most require a photo identification, and some require you to produce your original Social Security card, or furnish a copy. Your photo identification should be a government-issued document, such as a driver's license, state identification card, or passport. The name on the photo identification should be the same as the name used to register for the test, including suffixes such as "Jr.," "III," and the like. The photo identification card must also bear your signature. Each state has a list of acceptable identification that is given to candidates when they register for the test. If you do not have proper photo identification, contact the testing service well in advance to make arrangements for an alternate means of identification. Some states require two different forms of identification. Learn the requirements in advance and be prepared to meet them. In addition, some states require fingerprinting by a law enforcement agency prior to testing. It is the applicant's responsibility to see that this has been done in a timely manner, and to pay all associated fees. You may be required to bring the official (completed) fingerprint card with you at the time of testing. If you are late or fail to bring the required identification or supplies, you may not be admitted, so follow directions carefully.

You will not be permitted to bring audio or video recording devices or personal communication devices, such as pagers and cell phones, into the test site. Likewise, you may not bring children, visitors, or pets. (Service animals are not considered pets and will be admitted.) Do not bring valuables or weapons. You probably will not be permitted to take personal items other than your keys into the exam room. Leave purses, backpacks, books, notes, and other items in the car. You will not be permitted to eat, drink, or smoke during the examination. Students displaying disruptive behavior will be removed and the exam score recorded as a failure. If necessary, the skills examiner will call law enforcement authorities to remove or manage a disruptive candidate.

When you arrive at the test site, do not let another person's last-minute questions or comments upset you. Do not talk about the test to other students, if possible. Anxiety is contagious. Follow these general rules for taking the test:

1. Choose a good spot to sit. Make sure you have enough space. Maintain good posture and do not slouch. Be comfortable but alert. Stay relaxed and confident.

2. Remind yourself that you are well prepared and are going to do well. If you become anxious, take several slow, deep breaths to relax.

3. You will be given verbal instructions and be asked to complete an information form. Pay close attention to the examiner's instructions. He or she will read the directions. The examiner may not be permitted to answer questions.

4. Take several more deep breaths and try to relax. If you become anxious during the test, close your eyes for a few seconds and practice slow, deep breathing. Remaining relaxed and positive are keys to success. Remind yourself that you have studied well and are prepared to take the test. Think positive.

5. When you receive your test booklet, review the written directions and look at any sample questions. Make sure you understand how to mark your answers. Follow directions carefully. Most state tests are scored by computer, and stray marks will cause otherwise correct answers to be marked wrong. Write only on your answer sheet. Answers written in the exam book will not be counted.

6. Work at a steady pace.

7. Take the questions at face value. Do not read anything into them. Avoid thinking, "What if ?" Answer the question based on the information given. Do not look for tricks or hidden meanings. Do not add or subtract information.

8. Read the stem of the question. Think of the answer in your own words before reading the answers. Then read all the answers given. Search for the correct alternative, then select the option that most closely matches your answer. If necessary, read the stem with each option. If you are still not sure, treat each option as a true-false question, and choose the "most true."

9. It may be helpful to cross out unnecessary words in the question. Distracting information has been crossed out in this example:

   Q. A client ~~who~~ is HIV positive ~~understands that the nurse aide will not talk about this information outside the facility because~~ this information is

      a. legal.
      b. confidential.
      c. negligent.
      d. cultural.

10. If you do not know the answer to a question, circle the number and move on. Come back to it later. You may remember the answer later, or may find a clue to the answer in another question. Do not waste time struggling with questions you are unsure of. This increases your stress and test anxiety. Continuing with the test is best.

11. Be alert to words such as *not* and *except* that may completely change the intent of the question. Pay close attention to words that are *italicized*, CAPITALIZED, or are within "quotation marks" or (parentheses). Words such as *first*, *last*, *most*, *least*, *best*, and *except* often hold the key to the answer. Read carefully. These words are usually very important.

12. Avoid unfamiliar choices. Information that you are unfamiliar with is probably incorrect.

13. If you do not know the answer, try to determine what it is not. Cross out answers that you know or think are incorrect. If you have crossed out two answers, you have a 50% chance of guessing correctly. Other tips to help you:

    a. Question options that grammatically do not fit with the stem.
    b. Question options that are completely unfamiliar to you.
    c. Question options that contain negative or absolute words, such as those listed in number 11 above.
    d. Substitute a qualified term for the absolute one, such as "frequently" instead of "always." This may help you eliminate another incorrect answer.
    e. If two answers seem correct, compare them for differences, then refer to the stem to find your best answer.
    f. Use hints from questions that you know to help you answer questions that you do not.

14. Look at the shortest and longest of the remaining answers. The correct answer may be shorter or longer than the others.

15. There is no penalty for guessing. If you cannot figure out the answer, it is better to guess than to leave it blank.

16. Do not become upset or nervous if some individuals finish the test early and get up to leave. Some people read faster than others. Studies have shown that those who finish first do not necessarily get the best scores.

17. When you get to the end of the test, go back and complete the items you skipped.

18. Do not change your answers without a good reason. Your first answer is more likely to be correct. Change the answer if you misread or misunderstood the question, or if you are absolutely certain the first answer is wrong.

19. Before turning the test in, check it to make sure you marked every answer. Check the circles or boxes to be sure they are completely marked on the computer scoring sheet. Erase all stray marks.

MISCELLANEOUS TESTING CONCERNS

■ In some states, the written test is given on a computer. If you are taking a computerized test, you will be given several practice questions to make sure you know how to use the computer. Complete the practice questions. If you have difficulty with using the computer, speak with the skills examiner.

■ Some states administer oral examinations. Some states administer examinations in languages other than English. These special examinations must be requested from your state testing agency when you register to take the test. If you think you need an oral examination or non-English version of the test, contact your instructor or state testing service for information and instructions. The oral examinations are typically furnished on a cassette tape. You will listen to the tape with a head set. Typically, each question is read two times in a neutral manner. You will also be furnished with a written test booklet so you can review the printed words while listening to the tape. You will answer the question by marking the answer sheet. However, to be a nursing assistant, you must have the ability to read and write in English. Even if you will be taking an oral examination, you will be given a series of reading comprehension questions, typically 10. You must pass this portion of the examination, which shows your understanding of the English language, to pass the test. The time limits for oral testing are usually the same as the time limits for the written test.

■ Your state will accommodate individuals with certain disabilities during the test. Contact your state testing agency well in advance for information on requesting accommodations. You cannot wait until the day of the test to request a special accommodation.

■ Your state will have a skills (manual competency) examination portion of the state certification test. You must pass both portions of the test before you can be entered in the nursing assistant registry. Contact your instructor or state testing agency for information.

■ *Do not bring personal communication devices*, such as pagers, telephones, or other electronic devices, *to the test site. Use of these items will not be permitted.*

■ Do not give help to or receive help from anyone during the test. If the examiner suspects that a candidate is cheating on the examination, that person's test will be ended and the score recorded as a failure. You may be reported to your state nursing assistant registry for this activity.

■ Individuals caught removing a test from the testing site may be prosecuted. Copying, displaying, or distributing a copyrighted examination is illegal.

■ When you have finished testing, turn all paper materials in to the examiner. You may not remove the examination booklet, notes, or papers from the room.

THE SKILLS EXAMINATION

Part of the state test is a skills examination. This examination is administered slightly differently in each state. Usually, a nurse who has no affiliation with your school or educational program will administer the examination. You will be tested on the number of skills required by your state. Your skills will be chosen at random from the required skills list for your state. In most states, this is five skills. Reporting to the nurse, documenting, and doing basic calculations are parts of some skills. For example, if you weigh a resident, you must calculate the values of the upper and lower bars of the scale correctly. If you take a rectal or axillary temperature, you must show the skills examiner that you know how to record it correctly by placing an "R" or "A" after the temperature reading. If you count the pulse or respirations for 30 seconds, you must calculate and document the full-minute value correctly. If a value is abnormal, such as a temperature of 103.6° (R), you must recognize that the value is abnormal and report it to the nurse or proper person. If you empty a catheter bag or measure intake and output, you must use a graduate, measure, calculate, add, and document the total(s) correctly.

The passing rate for the skills component of the exam will vary with your state. Commonly, you must pass four or five skills to pass the examination. However, you need not complete each skill perfectly. Certain steps are designated as critical points in the skill. If you perform these correctly, you will pass the skill, even if you make a mistake. In some states, this testing is done in the skills laboratory using other students as resident volunteers. The examiner reads the student volunteer a statement and gives instructions on what is expected in playing the role of the resident. Treat the student volunteer exactly as you would a resident. Some skills, such as perineal care, may be done on a manikin. Pretend the manikin is a resident, and treat it with the same courtesy and precautions as you would use for a resident. All equipment and supplies will be available to perform the skill, but you must know what you need and gather it before beginning. Ask questions before you begin testing on the skill. Once the test begins, the nurse examiner will be unable to answer questions.

Some states do the skills test on residents in a nursing facility. Some states time the skills examination. For example, you are given 35 minutes in which to complete this portion of the test. Some states require you to pass the written test first, before you will be permitted to take the skills exam. In other states, the opposite is true. You must pass the skills examination before being permitted to take the written test. Although foreign language options are available for the written test, the skills examination is given only in English.

Preparing for the Skills Examination

The only way to adequately prepare for the skills examination is to practice each procedure in sequence. The skills that you will be tested on are randomly selected from the procedures you learned in class. If your nursing assistant class has a review day or mock skills examination before you take the test, be sure to attend. This will be very helpful to you in preparing for the test. You should also review your vocabulary terms so you are familiar with the various names for the procedures. For example, the skills examiner may direct you to "ambulate the resident." From your review of the vocabulary, you know that *ambulate* means to *walk*. If the examiner instructs you to do range of motion on the lower *extremities*, you must know that these are the *legs*. Practice your skills with other students or with your family, and use your procedure checklists or forms provided by your state. When reviewing the procedures, pay close attention to the list of supplies and equipment you will need to gather before you perform the procedure. It is essential that you collect the right supplies at the time of the skills test, or you may be unable to complete a procedure.

There is no way to study for the skills examination other than reviewing and practicing the procedures you have learned in class. The skills examiner will watch for some things during the examination. Some of these observations are very important and may be the deciding factor in whether you pass or fail a particular skill on the examination.

Observations Made During the Skills Examination

Gather all the supplies you will need before beginning each section of the test. If you will be making the bed, stack the linen in order of use. The test will go more smoothly if you are well organized.

Direct Care

Most of the skills examination consists of *direct care activities*. Direct resident care activities assist residents in meeting basic human needs, such as feeding, drinking, positioning, ambulating, grooming, toileting, and dressing. They may involve collecting, recording, and reporting information.

Indirect Care

Certain skills are part of every procedure you perform. These are usually called *indirect care skills*. Indirect activities focus on maintaining the environment and the systems in which nursing care is delivered. They assist in providing a clean, efficient, safe, comfortable, respectful resident care environment. An indirect care skill is an important part of the procedure, but does not necessarily affect the outcome. Data collection, documentation, consultation with other health care providers, and reporting information are indirect care skills. Examples of indirect care tasks are communication, comfort, resident rights, safety, and infection control. The skills examiner will look closely at (and score) your indirect care skills in each and every procedure. Doing these things each and every time is critical to your success. Indirect care skills on which you will be tested include the following essential elements:

- The skills examiner will observe *handwashing*. He or she will monitor your handwashing technique to be sure that you follow accepted standards and procedures. Wash your hands before and after caring for each resident, and more often as necessary. This skill will not be prompted by the examiner, meaning that you will not be told or reminded to do it. Nursing assistants are expected to know when and how to wash their hands. Use the proper technique. Each handwashing should last a minimum of 15 seconds, or according to your state rules.

- *Infection control* is another area on which you are evaluated. The skills examiner observes your technique in resident care, the use of standard precautions and medical asepsis. The examiner will also observe if you wear gloves and other PPE when necessary. You will be evaluated on whether you wash your hands before applying and removing gloves, as well as using proper technique in applying and removing the gloves themselves. Other important considerations are keeping clean and soiled items separated, disposing of soiled articles correctly, and preventing environmental contamination with used gloves and equipment.

- You will be observed in how well you *communicate* with each resident. You must introduce yourself and the skills examiner. Explain what you are going to do, even if the resident is confused. Inform the resident before each step, such as "Now I'm going to turn you over on your side." You may also be evaluated on whether you speak with the client throughout the procedure.

- The skills examiner will observe how well you practice *safety*. In fact, many safety violations constitute automatic test failures, such as leaving the bedside with the bed in the high position and side rails down. Another example is failure to lock the wheelchair brakes before transferring the resident. These are potentially serious problems that could result in resident injuries, and the skills examiners take them very seriously. Protect resident safety throughout the procedure. When you have finished the procedure, make sure the resident is left safe, with the call signal within reach. Do not leave the room if the resident is in an unsafe location or position, or if the ordered side rails or restraints are not in place.

- *Practicing resident rights* is also very important. Be sure to knock on doors and wait for permission to enter. Use the bath blanket for modesty when the resident's body will be exposed, such as during bathing and perineal care. Pull the privacy curtain, close the window curtains, and close the door to the room. Speak to the resident in a dignified manner. Avoid terms such as "honey," "dear," "granny," and "sweetie." Although facility staff may call residents by endearing names, the skills examiner will consider it undignified and unprofessional. Treat residents with the utmost respect at all times. The nurse examiner will monitor your attention to the resident's dignity, privacy, and safety.

- Resident *comfort* is an important consideration. You must ensure the residents' comfort by doing things such as handling the resident gently, asking about his or her comfort, supporting the arm when taking the blood pressure, positioning the resident in good body alignment, and leaving him or her in a comfortable position upon completion of the skill.

Critical Points

Critical points are things that could potentially harm a resident. If you skip a critical point on your state skills examination, you will fail the skill. If your state or program uses skills checklists with key or critical points listed, pay close attention to them. For example, in many states, failure to balance the scale before weighing a resident is a critical (automatic failure) point. Studying the critical points for each skill will be very helpful to you. Because these things could potentially harm a resident, you will feel more confident in providing care on the nursing units. Learning the critical points for each skill creates a win-win situation for both you and the residents. The following is an example of an actual skills test from one state. The underlined steps are the critical skills or automatic failure points.

Handwashing

1. Turns on water.

2. Wets hands.

3. Applies skin cleanser or soap to hands.

4. <u>Rubs hands together for at least 15 seconds in a circular motion.</u>

5. <u>Washes all surfaces of the hands at least up to the wrist.</u>

6. Rinses hands thoroughly from wrist to fingertips; cleans under fingernails, if needed; fingers down under running water.

7. Dries hands on clean towel/warm air dryer.

8. Turns off faucet with towel and/or <u>avoids contact with sink or other dirty surfaces during rinsing and drying of the hands.</u>

9. Discards wet towel appropriately.

When taking the skills test, think through each task that is asked of you. If the nurse examiner tells you that your resident has had a stroke with right-sided paralysis, then instructs you to get the resident out of bed, think about which side the resident will transfer to, where you will position the wheelchair, how you will keep the resident safe, and whether another assistant is needed to help. Critical points for this skill will include locking the wheelchair brakes and using a transfer belt (unless contraindicated).

Other Mistakes

If you think you have made a mistake or forget to do something during the skills examination, inform the skills examiner immediately. He or she may allow you to go back and correct the problem. This depends on the nature of the error and when you notify the examiner. If you inform the examiner of the error in a timely manner, he or she may permit you to go back and begin again at the point where the error was made. The skills examiner will not correct you if you make an error. He or she will not answer questions about the procedure during the test. If you have questions, ask them before testing begins. The skills examiner will not assist you or intervene during the test unless an unsafe resident condition develops.

AFTER THE TEST

After the test, you will breathe a sigh of relief. Listen carefully to the examiner's instructions for returning test materials. Information may also be provided about how and when you will find out the test results. In many states, you know the preliminary results the same day. You will not be given a percentage or letter grade. Preliminary scores are listed as either "pass" or "fail." The results are considered preliminary until they are validated by the testing agency in their offices. After the tests are validated, you will be given a more complete explanation of your score. You should receive a report in the mail in approximately two weeks. If you have not received the results within 30 days, contact the examination service.

If you have passed the written and skills examinations, your name will be entered into your state nursing assistant registry. This may take several weeks. In some states, the criminal background and fingerprint checks must also be cleared before you are entered into the registry. You will be issued a wallet card to show your employer as proof of your certification. Protect your wallet card and do not lose it. Never give your employer or a prospective employer the original. If they need a copy, make a photocopy and keep the original in a safe place. If you lose your card, your state will issue a duplicate, but there is usually a fee for this service. Your certification must be current for the state to issue a duplicate card. Do not alter your card in any way. Altering the card may result in loss of certification.

If you did not pass the test, you will have at least two more opportunities to retest. You have three opportunities to pass each part of the examination. However, there is a fee for each retesting. Your instructor must register you for the retest. All testing fees must be submitted to the testing service at the time of registration. Meet with your instructor to find out what to study to increase your chances of successfully passing the retest.

You must keep your state nursing assistant registry informed of any changes in your name or address. If you move or change your name, notify the state registry promptly in writing. Provide them with your state registration number or Social Security number so the information can be listed for the proper person. (More than one person may have the same name.) Many states have forms available on their Web sites to submit for change of name or address.

Your nursing assistant certification will expire in 24months. To renew it, you must meet your state continuing education requirements. To remain active, you must submit a form verifying that you have provided nursing assistant services during the renewal period. The number of hours you are required to work to maintain your certification varies with each state.

PART IV

Documentation and Forms

NURSING ASSISTANT DOCUMENTATION

THE MEDICAL RECORD

Each health care facility must maintain clinical records on each resident, following accepted professional health information management standards. Documentation is the validation of quality care. Your instructor will stress that your job is not done until you have documented the care you gave.

All health status data about the resident must be available for all members of the health care team. The resident's medical records should be accessible, communicated, and recorded. Because all team members depend on the information in the medical record, documentation is a big responsibility. The record must be honest, objective, accurate, and complete. It must reflect the use of the nursing process, and show that the resident received care that met minimum acceptable standards.

The adage, "If it was not documented, it was not done," is as valid today as it was 50 years ago. In years past, some nurses thought that care was the main priority and documentation was secondary. Today, we cannot choose between giving care and keeping records. Both are important. The medical record and documentation are part of the resident's care, and validation of that care. Without accurate and complete documentation, no one knows with certainty what has been done. If the record is incomplete or inaccurate, it is difficult for caregivers to set goals or plan future clinical approaches to the resident's care. When the record is completely documented, it provides

- the information needed to plan care.
- the information needed to ensure continuity of care.
- a means of communication among team members.
- written evidence of the rationale for treatments and care given.
- proof of modification of the care plan, the resident's response to the plan, and whether the plan was effective.
- a means of monitoring resident care on an ongoing basis.
- a vehicle for review, study, and evaluation of resident care.
- a legal record that protects the resident, facility, and health care personnel.
- a means of identifying and communicating information about the residents' problems, needs, and strengths.

LEGAL EVIDENCE

Documentation is a legal record of the resident's care. As a legal document, the medical record can be used in a court of law. The notes are admitted as legal evidence. Lawyers, judges, juries, experts, and others may read them. If a medical record is used in a trial, the documentation shows that care was or was not given. This affects the outcome of the trial. When a note from the chart is used in a lawsuit, the worker who wrote the note may also have to testify at the trial. Testifying is a frightening, stressful experience. Lawsuits move very slowly through the courts. They often go to trial several years after care was given. You may not remember exactly what you did. Your notes must be complete to prove what you did. Thorough notes help you defend your actions.

Your charting should leave no question in a reader's mind that you provided needed care and monitored residents' conditions. Tampering with, falsifying, altering, or destroying data in a resident's chart is illegal and unethical. One falsification can call the credibility of the entire record into question. By extension, the credibility and integrity of the personnel who documented in the record may also be questioned. Personnel may be charged with fraud based on falsification of records and documention of care that was not provided. Charting in advance is also falsification. The only part of the record that may be documented in advance is the care plan. All other data are charted after being done.

Accountability

Everyone who cares for residents is responsible for documentation. Each worker is responsible for documenting the services he or she provides. Health care workers cannot document for each other. Each worker is responsible for what he or she has written. Every entry in the chart is evidence that care was given. You cannot document care that you did not provide. For example, you know you must turn and reposition a resident every two hours. You will document that you turned the resident every two hours because you *actually did it*, not because it is care that is *supposed to be given*.

Surveys

Surveyors review documentation when they visit the facility. Complete, accurate documentation proves that workers have complied with the law. It shows that the residents have received good care. The record should show that the residents' risks and needs were identified, and that care was given to meet those needs. Missing or absent documentation commonly results in deficiencies. Surveyors may ask questions about information in the chart. However, you should view documentation as something that helps care for the resident. It is much more than paper compliance.

DOCUMENTATION FORMAT

Most long-term care facilities use a system called *source-oriented medical records (SOMR)*. The information in the SOMR is divided into categories. Each discipline has a separate divider in the chart in which their records are stored. The sequence of the record varies from one facility to the next.

Some facilities use the *problem-oriented medical record (POMR)*. This type of record is divided into five general categories, and all disciplines chart in each category. Facilities that use this system believe it improves communication. They state that it makes finding information easier.

Many different formats are used for recording information on the medical record. Medications, treatments, and ADLs are recorded on flow sheets. The caregiver initials a box, showing that care was given. Two other common formats are the *narrative format* and *SOAP documentation*. Facilities that use the narrative format describe the resident's care like a story. SOAP is an abbreviation for Subjective, Objective, Assessment, Plan. Facilities using this format write an entry for each category. For example:

- *S* stands for subjective. Because symptoms are subjective findings, they are described in this section. The resident, family member, or caregiver provides the information.

- *O* stands for objective. The information here is based on observations by the caregiver. The signs of the resident's condition are recorded in this section. Information about the resident's ability to function also goes in this section.

- *A* stands for assessment. The nurse practice act in most states prohibits unlicensed caregivers from assessing residents. However, you will assist with assessments by collecting information such as vital signs. You report your findings to a licensed professional. Because assessment is a professional responsibility, you must be careful about wording information in this section. You may want to think of the "A" here as an abbreviation for an analysis. You are not permitted to assess, so write your analysis of the situation.

- *P* stands for plan. The plan describes the treatment information. You will document care listed in the plans for each resident.

Another popular system similar to SOAP is the *APIE system*. This meaning of this abbreviation is

- *A* = assessment

- *P* = plan

- *I* = implementation of the plan

- *E* = evaluation of the resident's response to the plan

Some facilities use a documentation system called *charting by exception (CBE)*. In this system, normal findings and routine care are not documented. Only abnormals are documented. CBE is a formal system with policies, procedures, and special forms. It is not an informal method of documentation used because staff forgets to document. Exceptions to expected observations are always charted. Many facilities believe this is a risky method of charting, because it does not provide legal proof that care was given. Some facilities have had difficulty getting reimbursed for care without documentation to verify that the care was given.

DOCUMENTING IN THE MEDICAL RECORD

Follow your facility policies and your state's legal guidelines for documentation. Most facilities have a policy for using colored ink in the medical record. Chart only in the accepted color. Many facilities use only black, because it is clear and copies well. Avoid using erasable or nonpermanent ink. Remember that the medical record is a legal document that will be read by others. The information must always be accurate. Never record care that you did not give. Avoid making up or overstating information.

Avoid providing the opportunity for the record to be altered. For example, notes written in pencil or erasable ink can be changed. Do not use these instruments to write on medical records. Avoid leaving blank lines. These provide space for someone to change the record. If there are blank spaces, draw a line through them. This prevents others from filling them in. Never try to erase, obliterate, or white out an error. If you make an error, follow your facility policy for correcting it. In most facilities, you will draw a single line through the entry. Write the word "error" next to or above the entry. Sign the changes. Keep your documentation brief and concise.

Abbreviations

Use only acceptable, recognized abbreviations. Abbreviations are easily misunderstood. Some have more than one meaning. Limit the use of abbreviations and make sure that you use the accepted ones correctly. You will use some standard nursing abbreviations in your documentation. Many abbreviations are listed in the main text. This was done so that you could learn to understand documentation and have a resource for checking information you see in medical records and other documents in your facility. Your facility will have a specific list of abbreviations to use in your charting. *Use only abbreviations that your facility accepts and recognizes.*

JCAHO has approved a "minimum list" of dangerous abbreviations, acronyms, and symbols. These abbreviations may be misunderstood and thus increase the risk of errors. Beginning January 1, 2004, accredited facilities must include certain items on their "do not use" lists. Of the abbreviations listed, the following are commonly used for nursing assistant documentation:

- Q.D., Q.O.D. (Latin abbreviation for once daily and every other day)

The JCAHO requires facilities to periodically add other abbreviations to the "do not use" list. They recommend these for subsequent elimination from approved lists:

- H.S. (for half-strength or Latin abbreviation for bedtime)

- T.I.W. (for three times a week)

- D/C (for discharge)

- c.c. (for cubic centimeter)

The Institute for Safe Medication Practices has also updated its list of unsafe abbreviations. They recommend that the following be removed from use:

- OD (right eye)
- ʒ (dram)
- OJ (orange juice)
- per os (by mouth)
- qhs (nightly at bedtime)
- > < (greater than and less than)
- @ (at)
- & (and)
- + (plus or and)
- ° (hour)

Frequency of Documentation

A record is made each time you care for a resident. At the very least, you will initial a box on a flow sheet. You may be required to write a special note about an unusual situation, significant improvement, or decline. Always document if the resident refuses treatment. If you are documenting a refusal on a flow sheet, place an "R" in the box. Explain the refusal on the back of the record.

Timeliness of Documentation

Document your care in a timely manner. Never chart before providing care. Document as soon as possible after caring for the resident. Sometimes you cannot document immediately after caring for the resident, so carry a small notebook. Record important information that you can transfer to your notes later. If you forget to document something, and then remember later, follow facility policy for late entry documentation. Usually, you will write the date and time the entry is made. You will begin the entry by writing, "Late entry for (date, time)."

Understanding the Information

Your documentation must be clear to anyone who reads the chart. Your entries must be legible. Illegible information is easily misinterpreted. When documenting on flow sheets, make sure you use the correct box. If your handwriting is not legible, print. Your punctuation, grammar, and spelling must be correct. An accurate and concise record shows that you are conscientious. It implies that you have given quality care. Errors suggest that you are careless. If you are careless with your documentation, the reader may assume that you are careless with the care you give.

Signing the Entry

Follow your facility policy for signing each entry. Some facilities require you to sign your complete legal signature. Others use the first initial and last name. Your title and/or certification follow your name. Flow sheets will have a key for the initials. Make sure you sign the key each month so others can identify your entries. Do not sign a flow sheet unless you are responsible for documenting on it.

As you can see, documentation is a key element of the care you give. It is not something you do strictly to satisfy regulations. Accurate, complete documentation benefits the residents and protects you legally. It proves that you gave quality, conscientious care.

DOCUMENTATION EXERCISES

CLINICAL SITUATION: CARING FOR MR. BARANYI

Mr. Henry Baranyi was admitted to your facility on May 31 for rehabilitation following an acute hospital stay for a stroke. He has left-sided paralysis. He has a history of congestive heart failure. He retains fluid when he is up, but puts out large amounts at night when he is in bed. His height is 68", weight 146#, and vital signs 98.2°F (O) - 68 - 16 - 144/96. This 75-year-old widower has lived alone since his wife died 10 years ago. Before the stroke, he lived in a small house, and took great pleasure in tending his flower garden. He drove a car and went to the senior center daily. He hopes to return home and use a home health assistant.

Mr. Baranyi can speak and make his needs known, but is forgetful. He is incontinent of urine and stool. He feeds himself after tray setup. The nurse schedules him for breakfast in his room, and lunch and dinner in the main dining room. He is on a low-sodium diet. He wears glasses and hears normally. He needs assistance with bathing, dressing, and grooming. He has his own teeth, which are in good repair. His skin is dry and fragile. He is scheduled for a whirlpool bath on the day shift Monday, Wednesday, and Friday. He transfers with a transfer belt with one assistant. He needs a lap buddy when in the wheelchair to remind him not to get up alone. The resident can turn to the left, but needs assistance turning to the right when in bed. His bed has four half rails. The two upper rails are raised to help the resident with turning. The hospital reports that he has never tried to get out of bed without help. The two lower side rails are down when he is in bed, and the nurse says they will evaluate his bed safety. The nurse asked him about a numeric (1 to 10) pain scale, but he did not seem to understand the numbers. The resident is frustrated because of his loss of independence.

The resident brought the following items to the facility: 4 sweat pants, 4 slacks, 10 shirts, 10 t-shirts, 8 boxer shorts, 12 pairs socks, 1 pair sneakers, 1 pair slippers, 2 pairs pajamas, 1 robe, 1 color TV with remote control, comb, brush, deodorant, electric razor, eyeglasses, toothbrush, toothpaste. His daughter said she would bring some additional items later.

Mr. Baranyi has orders for TED hose when out of bed, PROM T.I.D., PT daily, an OT evaluation for self-help skills, and a nursing assessment for bowel and bladder retraining. The doctor has ordered intake and output monitoring, weekly weight, and vital signs daily.

DOCUMENTATION ACTIVITIES

Ask your instructor to duplicate the forms in this section, if needed. Complete the documentation activities based on your knowledge of Mr. Baranyi's history and physician orders and the care in the following list. Use the forms in your workbook, or facility forms provided by your instructor. The resident's assigned medical record number is R93638.

Activity 1
Complete the nursing assistant care plan for Mr. Baranyi. Start the June ADL sheet, restraint record, and a bowel and bladder assessment by filling in the relevant information from the history and physician orders.

Activity 2
Complete the resident's admission forms. Complete the personal inventory form.

Activity 3
Monday, June 1—You are assigned to care for Mr. Baranyi on the 6:00 a.m. to 2:00 p.m. shift. Complete the nursing assistant communication log and ADL sheet for your shift. Select the correct forms and document the following care:

Vital signs: 97.4°F (O) - 64 - 16 - 132/88

Intake 1140 mL; Output—incontinent of urine x 3

Had a moderate BM (incontinent)

B&B monitoring: 6:00 a.m. wet large, 7:00 a.m. dry, 8:00 a.m. dry, 9:00 a.m. dry, 10:00 a.m. wet small and mod BM, 11:00 a.m. dry, 12:00 p.m. dry, 1:00 p.m. wet large, 2:00 p.m. dry

Appetite breakfast: 100%

Appetite lunch: 85%

Bath: whirlpool with shampoo

Oral care: assist

Shave: self with electric razor

Nail care: nails cleaned

Linen change: complete

Activity: up in wheelchair with cushion to prevent skin breakdown

Turned q2h in bed, repositioned q1h in w/c

Exercise: PROM x 2

Restraints: side rails x 2 in bed, lap buddy in chair

Bathing in whirlpool: self with one assist

Body alignment: self limited; one assist

Dressing: self with one assist

Toileting: dependent on staff

Grooming: self with one assist

Ambulation: dependent on staff

Transfers: self with one assist

Eating: self with setup

Activity 4

Tuesday, June 2—You are assigned to care for Mr. Baranyi on the 6:00 a.m. to 2:00 p.m. shift. Complete the nursing assistant communication log and ADL sheet for your shift. Select the correct forms and document the following care:

Vital signs: 97.2°F (O) - 60 - 16 - 132/86

Intake 1260 mL; Output—incontinent of urine x 3

Moderate BM (incontinent)

B&B monitoring: 6:00 a.m. dry, 7:00 a.m. dry, 8:00 a.m. incontinent large urine and mod BM, 9:00 a.m. dry, 10:00 a.m. dry, 11:00 a.m. dry, 12:00 p.m. incontinent large, 1:00 p.m. dry, 2:00 p.m. dry

Appetite breakfast: 90%

Appetite lunch: 100%

Bath: PBB

Oral care: assist

Shave: self with electric razor

Linen change: partial

Activity: up in wheelchair with cushion to prevent skin breakdown

Turned q2h in bed, repositioned q1h in w/c

Exercise: PROM x 2

Restraints: side rails x 2 in bed, lap buddy in chair

Partial bath: self with one assist

Body alignment: self limited; one assist

Dressing: self with one assist

Toileting: dependent on staff

Grooming: self with one assist

Ambulation: dependent on staff

Transfers: self with one assist

Eating: self with setup

Activity 5

Wednesday, June 3—You are assigned to care for Mr. Baranyi on the 6:00 a.m. to 2:00 p.m. shift. Complete the ADL sheet for your shift. Fill out a form with information you will turn in to the nurse at the end of the shift. Select the correct forms and document the following care:

Vital signs: 98.6°F (O) - 70 - 16 - 148/92

Intake 980 mL; Output—incontinent of urine x 2

Large BM (incontinent)

B&B monitoring: 6:00 a.m. dry, 7:00 a.m. dry, 8:00 a.m. dry, 9:00 a.m. incontinent large urine and BM, 10:00 a.m. dry, 11:00 a.m. dry, 12:00 p.m. dry, 1:00 p.m. incontinent large, 2:00 p.m. dry

Appetite breakfast: 80%

Appetite lunch: 40%, accepted substitute and ate 90% of it

Bath: whirlpool with shampoo

Oral care: assist

Shave: self with electric razor

Nail care: nails cleaned

Linen change: complete

Activity: up in wheelchair with cushion to prevent skin breakdown

Turned q2h in bed, repositioned q1h in w/c

Exercise: PROM x 2

Restraints: side rails x 2 in bed, lap buddy in chair

Bathing in whirlpool: self with one assist

Body alignment: self limited; one assist

Dressing: self with one assist

Toileting: dependent on staff

Grooming: self with one assist

Ambulation: dependent on staff

Transfers: self with one assist

Eating: self with setup

Activity 6

Thursday, June 4—You are assigned to care for Mr. Baranyi on the 6:00 a.m. to 2:00 p.m. shift. Complete the ADL sheet for your shift. Fill out a form with information you will turn in to the nurse at the end of the shift. Select the correct forms and document the following care:

Vital signs: 97.8°F (O) - 74 - 14 - 140/82

Intake 1190 mL; Output—incontinent x 4

No BM

B&B monitoring: 6:00 a.m. wet large, 7:00 a.m. dry, 8:00 a.m. wet small, 9:00 a.m. dry, 10:00 a.m. dry, 11:00 a.m. wet moderate, 12:00 p.m. dry, 1:00 p.m. dry, 2:00 p.m. wet large

Appetite breakfast: 75%

Appetite lunch: 100%

Bath: whirlpool with shampoo

Oral care: assist

Shave: self with electric razor

Linen change: complete

Activity: up in wheelchair with cushion to prevent skin breakdown

Turned q2h in bed, repositioned q1h in w/c

Exercise: PROM x 2

Restraints: side rails x 2 in bed, lap buddy in chair

Partial bath: self with one assist

Body alignment: self limited; one assist

Dressing: self with one assist
Toileting: dependent on staff
Grooming: self with one assist
Ambulation: dependent on staff
Transfers: self with one assist
Eating: self with setup

Activity 7

Monday, June 8—You are assigned to care for Mr. Baranyi on the 6:00 a.m. to 2:00 p.m. shift. Complete the ADL sheet for your shift. Select the correct forms and document the following care:

Vital signs: 98°F (O) - 80 - 20 - 146/88
Weight: 140
Intake 1040 mL; Output—incontinent x 3
Had a moderate BM (incontinent)
B&B monitoring: 6:00 a.m. dry, 7:00 a.m. wet large, 8:00 a.m. dry, 9:00 a.m. dry, 10:00 a.m. wet large urine, incontinent mod BM, 11:00 a.m. dry, 12:00 p.m. dry, 1:00 p.m. wet small, 2:00 p.m. dry
Appetite breakfast: 60%, refused substitute
Appetite lunch: 90%
House shake at 10:00 a.m. and 2:00 p.m.: new order 10:00 a.m. not given, 2:00 p.m. consumed 100%
Bath: whirlpool with shampoo
Oral care: assist
Shave: self with electric razor
Nail care: nails cleaned
Linen change: partial
Activity: up in wheelchair with cushion to prevent skin breakdown
Turned q2h in bed, repositioned q1h in w/c
Exercise: PROM x 2
Restraints: side rails x 2 in bed, lap buddy in chair
The dietitian evaluated the resident and noted that he was at the low end of his ideal body weight range of 139 to 169 pounds. She recommended giving the resident a house shake at 10:00 a.m., 2:00 p.m., and bedtime. She also recommended that he be given a sandwich at bedtime. The nurse instructs you to begin giving the shakes today, and reminds you to document his intake.

Activity 8

Tuesday, June 9—You are assigned to care for Mr. Baranyi on the 6:00 a.m. to 2:00 p.m. shift. Complete the ADL sheet for your shift. Fill out a form with information you will turn in to the nurse at the end of the shift. Select the correct forms and document the following care:
Vital signs: 98.8°F (O) - 60 - 14 - 132/84
Intake 1320 mL; Output—incontinent of urine x 4
Had a moderate BM (incontinent)
B&B monitoring: 6:00 a.m. wet large, 7:00 a.m. dry, 8:00 a.m. wet small, 9:00 a.m. dry, 10:00 a.m. dry, 11:00 a.m. wet moderate and mod BM, 12:00 p.m. dry, 1:00 p.m. wet small, 2:00 p.m. dry
Appetite breakfast: 90%
Appetite lunch: 85%
House shake at 10:00 a.m.: 80%
House shake at 2:00 p.m.: 100%
Bath: whirlpool with shampoo
Oral care: assist
Shave: self with electric razor
Linen change: partial
Activity: up in wheelchair with cushion to prevent skin breakdown

Turned q2h in bed, repositioned q1h in w/c
Exercise: PROM x 2
Restraints: side rails x 2 in bed, lap buddy in chair
The nurse reminds you to attend the resident's care conference. She reminds you to bring the completed seven-day self-ability evaluation form. You were responsible for documenting on this form on June 1, 2, 3, and 4.

Activity 9

Wednesday, June 10—You are assigned to care for Mr. Baranyi on the 6:00 a.m. to 2:00 p.m. shift. Complete the ADL sheet for your shift. Fill out a form with information you will turn in to the nurse at the end of the shift. Select the correct forms and document the following care:

Vital signs: 98.4°F (O) - 70 - 16 - 140/82
Intake 1220 mL; Output—incontinent of urine x 2, 200 mL in urinal
Had a small BM (requested to use toilet)
B&B monitoring: 6:00 a.m. wet large, 7:00 a.m. dry, 8:00 a.m. dry, 9:00 a.m. dry, 10:00 a.m. 200 in urinal, 11:00 a.m. dry, 12:00 p.m. dry, 1:00 p.m. incontinent moderate, 2:00 p.m. dry, asked to use toilet for BM—did not void.
Appetite breakfast: 100%
Appetite lunch: 100%
House shake at 10:00 a.m.: 100%
House shake at 2:00 p.m.: 100%
Bath: whirlpool with shampoo
Oral care: assist
Shave: self with electric razor
Nail care: nails cleaned
Linen change: partial
Activity: up in wheelchair with cushion to prevent skin breakdown
Turned q2h in bed, repositioned q1h in w/c
Exercise: PROM x 2
Restraints: side rails x 2 in bed, lap buddy in chair

Mr. Baranyi's daughter brings some additional personal items. Add these items to his personal inventory: 1 denim jacket, a blue sweater that zips up the front, a red pullover sweater, a Timex wristwatch with a black band, a clock radio, a worn black Bible, a rosary, a photo album, a blue-and-white lap blanket that she had crocheted, and a blue quilted bedspread.

Activity 10

Thursday, June 11—You are assigned to care for Mr. Baranyi on the 6:00 a.m. to 2:00 p.m. shift. Complete the ADL sheet for your shift. Fill out a form with information you will turn in to the nurse at the end of the shift. Select the correct forms and document the following care:

Vital signs: 98.6°F (O) - 68 - 18 - 142/82
Intake 1156 mL; Output—incontinent of urine x 2, urinal 230 mL x 1, urine-150 mL, toilet x 1
Had a moderate BM (requested to use toilet)
B&B monitoring: 6:00 a.m. urinal 230 mL, 7:00 a.m. dry, 8:00 a.m. incontinent moderate, 9:00 a.m. dry, 10:00 a.m. dry, 11:00 a.m. incontinent small, 12:00 p.m. dry, 1:00 p.m. toilet 150 mL and moderate BM, 2:00 p.m. dry
Appetite breakfast: 85%
Appetite lunch: 95%
House shake at 10:00 a.m.: 75%
House shake at 2:00 p.m.: 100%
Bath: PBB
Oral care: assist

Shave: self with electric razor
Linen change: complete
Activity: up in wheelchair with cushion to prevent skin breakdown
Turned q2h in bed, repositioned q1h in w/c
Exercise: PROM x 2
Restraints: side rails x 2 in bed, lap buddy in chair

Activity 11

Friday, June 12—You are assigned to care for Mr. Baranyi on the 6:00 a.m. to 2:00 p.m. shift. Complete the ADL sheet for your shift. Fill out a form with information you will turn in to the nurse at the end of the shift. Select the correct forms and document the following care:

Vital signs: 98.4°F (O) - 68 - 16 - 148/80
Intake 1288 mL; Output—incontinent of urine x 2, urinal 220 mL
Had a large BM (incontinent)
B&B monitoring: 6:00 a.m. dry, 7:00 a.m. incontinent moderate urine and large BM, 8:00 a.m. dry, 9:00 a.m.
    dry, 10:00 a.m. dry, 11:00 a.m. urinal 220 mL, 12:00 p.m. dry, 1:00 p.m. dry, 2:00 p.m. wet moderate
Appetite breakfast: 100%
Appetite lunch: 100%
House shake at 10:00 a.m.: 80%
House shake at 2:00 p.m.: 50%
Bath: whirlpool with shampoo
Oral care: assist
Shave: self with electric razor
Linen change: partial
Activity: up in wheelchair with cushion to prevent skin breakdown
Turned q2h in bed, repositioned q1h in w/c
Exercise: PROM x 2
Restraints: side rails x 2 in bed, lap buddy in chair

Activity 12

Monday, June 15—You are assigned to care for Mr. Baranyi on the 6:00 a.m. to 2:00 p.m. shift. Complete the ADL sheet for your shift. Fill out a form with information you will turn in to the nurse at the end of the shift. Select the correct forms and document the following care:

Vital signs: 97.2°F (O) - 60 - 14 - 154/88
Weight: 143
Intake 1066 mL; Output—incontinent of urine x 1, urinal x 2
No BM.
B&B monitoring: 6:00 a.m. dry, 7:00 a.m. urinal 176 mL, 8:00 a.m. dry, 9:00 a.m. dry, 10:00 a.m. wet small,
    11:00 a.m. dry, 12:00 p.m. dry, 1:00 p.m. urinal 272 mL, 2:00 p.m. dry
Appetite breakfast: 80%
Appetite lunch: 90%
House shake at 10:00 a.m.: 100%
House shake at 2:00 p.m.: 90%
Bath: whirlpool with shampoo
Oral care: assist
Shave: self with electric razor
Linen change: complete
Activity: up in wheelchair with cushion to prevent skin breakdown
Turned q2h in bed, repositioned q1h in w/c
Exercise: PROM x 2
Restraints: side rails x 2 in bed, lap buddy in chair

Activity 13

Tuesday, June 16—You are assigned to care for Mr. Baranyi on the 6:00 a.m. to 2:00 p.m. shift. Complete the ADL sheet for your shift. Select the correct forms and document the following care:

Vital signs: 98.4°F (O) - 70 - 16 - 128/86

Intake 1236 mL; Output—incontinent of urine x 1, urinal x 2, toilet x 1

Small BM (toilet)

B&B monitoring: 6:00 a.m. wet moderate, 7:00 a.m. 180 mL urinal, 8:00 a.m. dry, 9:00 a.m. dry, 10:00 a.m. 264 mL urinal, 11:00 a.m. dry, 12:00 p.m. dry, 1:00 p.m. dry, 2:00 p.m. 248 mL toilet and small BM.

Appetite breakfast: 70%, refused substitute

Appetite lunch: 80%

House shake at 10:00 a.m.: 50%

House shake at 2:00 p.m.: 70%

Bath: PBB

Oral care: assist

Shave: self with electric razor

Nail care: nails cleaned

Linen change: partial

Activity: up in wheelchair with cushion to prevent skin breakdown

Turned q2h in bed, repositioned q1h in w/c

Exercise: PROM x 2

Restraints: side rails x 2 in bed, lap buddy in chair

Activity 14

Wednesday, June 17—You are assigned to care for Mr. Baranyi on the 6:00 a.m. to 2:00 p.m. shift. Complete the nursing assistant communication log and ADL sheet for your shift. Select the correct forms and document the following care:

Vital signs: 98.6°F (O) - 76 - 18 - 150/94

Intake 1322 mL; Output—incontinent of urine x 1, urinal x 2, toilet x 1

No BM

B&B monitoring: 6:00 a.m. urinal 274 mL, 7:00 a.m. dry, 8:00 a.m. dry, 9:00 a.m. incontinent small, 10:00 a.m. dry, 11:00 a.m. dry, 12:00 p.m. urinal 300 mL, 1:00 p.m. dry, 2:00 p.m. toilet 238 mL

Appetite breakfast: 80%

Appetite lunch: 100%

House shake at 10:00 a.m.: 100%

House shake at 2:00 p.m.: 100%

Bath: whirlpool with shampoo

Oral care: assist

Shave: self with electric razor

Nail care: nails cleaned

Linen change: complete

Activity: up in wheelchair with cushion to prevent skin breakdown

Turned q2h in bed, repositioned q1h in w/c

Exercise: PROM x 2

Restraints: side rails x 2 in bed, lap buddy in chair

FORMS FOR DOCUMENTATION

Nursing Assistant Care Plan
ADL Flow Sheets
Intake-Output Worksheets
Resident Restraint Records
Documentation of Meal Intake
Initial Incontinence Evaluation (Voiding Pattern Assessment)
Assessment for Bowel and Bladder Training
Weight Record
Vital Sign Record
Graphic Record
Inventory of Personal Effects
Seven-Day Resident Self-Ability Evaluation
Resident Care Worksheet
Nursing Assistant Assignment Sheet

NURSING ASSISTANT CARE PLAN

DIETARY

Diabetic _____ Calorie ☐

Dining Room: Bkfst. Lunch Dinner

Room: Bkfst. Lunch Dinner

Feeder Room: Bkfst. Lunch Dinner

Set Tray Up ☐

Feed ☐

Tube Feeding ☐

Adaptive Equipment

_____
Diet

_____
Nourishment/Supplement/HS Snack

Measure:

Intake ☐

Output ☐

ELIMINATION

Toilet q 2 hrs. ☐

Bedpan/Urinal ☐

Incontinence Bowel ☐

Incontinence Bladder ☐

Catheter

Foley ☐

Supra Pubic ☐

Condom ☐

Leg Bag ☐

Catheter Strap ☐

Ostomy ☐

BATHING

Tub ☐

Shower ☐

Bed ☐

Day: M T W T F S S

AM ☐   PM ☐

Shampoo

Beauty Shop ☐

Staff ☐

AM/PM Care

Self ☐

Staff ☐

Shave by Noon, Remove Facial Hair. Finger Nail Care on Bath/Shower Day. Toe Nail Care as Directed by Nurse.

HEARING

Hard of Hearing:

Right ☐ Left ☐

Hearing Aid:

Right ☐ Left ☐

Look at Resident While Speaking to Them.

FREQUENCY OF VITAL SIGNS

Weight _____

TPR _____

B/P _____

POSITIONING

Turn q 2 hours ☐

Range of Motion with Cares ☐

Special Mattress/Device

_____

Positioning Equip.

_____

Braces/Splints/Cones

_____

Follow Turning Schedule.

DRESSING

Self ☐

Assist ☐

Supervise ☐

Total ☐

Adult Brief ☐

Lap robe ☐

All Residents to Wear Underwear.

SIGHT

Blind:

Right ☐ Left ☐

Poor Vision ☐

Glasses ☐

Contact Lens ☐

Clean Glasses or Contact Lens with A.M. Care.

ORAL CARE

Self ☐

Assist ☐

Own Teeth ☐

No Teeth ☐

Dentures:

Upper ☐

Lower ☐

Partial ☐

Oral Care in A.M., at Bedtime and PRN.

MOBILITY

Independent ☐

Cane ☐

Walker ☐

Wheelchair ☐

Own ☐

Other ☐

No Weight Bearing:

Right ☐ Left ☐

Partial Weight Bearing

Right ☐ Left ☐

Gait Belt ☐

Transfer ☐

Hoyer Lift ☐

No. of Assist for Transfers

_____

Other _____

RESTRAINTS

Vest: When _____ ☐

Waist (soft) When in Chair ☐

Mitts _____ ☐

Geri Chair ☐

Roller Bar: When in W/C ☐

Lap Belt ☐

Other _____ ☐

Restrain at All Times ☐

SIDERAILS

At All Times ☐

At Night Only ☐

Signed Release: ☐

Do not use any restraint not checked above. Observe q 30 minutes and release q 2 hours x's 10 minutes for care/exercise.

Special Instructions: _____
_____
_____
_____
_____
_____
_____
_____
_____
_____
_____
_____
_____

Room No.: _____   Date: _____

Resident: _____

ADL FLOWSHEET

Category	Sub	HR	1	2	3	4	5	6	7	8	9	10	11	12	13	14	15	16	17	18	19	20	21	22	23	24	25	26	27	28	29	30	31
Diet: 75% (GOOD) 50% (FAIR) 25% (POOR) R-Refused		B																															
( ) DINING ROOM S = SUBSTITUTE		L																															
( ) ROOM ( ) ASSISTANCE ( ) TOTAL		D																															
( ) FEEDS SELF		S																															
Bath		D																															
( ) Bed Bath (BB) ( ) Whirlpool (WP) ( ) Independent (I) ( ) Shower (SH) ( ) Assisted (A) ( ) Tub Bath (TB) ( ) Partial Bath (PB) ( ) Total Help (TH)		E																															
Oral Care ( ) Independent (I)		N																															
( ) Dentures ( ) Assisted (A)		D																															
( ) Teeth ( ) Total Help (TH)		E																															
Fingernail Care ( ) I ( ) A ( ) TH		N																															
Toenail Care ( ) I ( ) A ( ) TH		N																															
Shave ( ) I ( ) A ( ) TH		S																															
Shampoo ( ) I ( ) A ( ) TH		S																															
Bowel Movement (BM) M = Medium		N																															
S = Small O = None		D																															
L = Large		E																															
( ) Incontinent (I) (Check Only One) ( ) Continent (C)		N																															
( ) Urine		D																															
( ) Peri-care after each incontinent episode		E																															
( ) Incontinent (I) (Check Only One) ( ) Continent (C)		N																															
( ) Feces		D																															
( ) Sponge bath after each incontinent episode		E																															
Skin Care ( ) Turn and reposition Q2h		N																															
( ) Peri-care		D																															
( ) Back rub		E																															
Ambulation ( ) Partial Bedfast ( ) Independent		N																															
( ) Walker ( ) Geri-chair ( ) Assistant ( ) AMB ( ) Wheelchair ( ) Total Help		D																															
( ) Cane		E																															
Protective Safety Device Q 1 hr, R/R Q 2 hrs × 10 min.		N																															
( ) Vest ( ) Side Rails		D																															
( ) Waist ( ) Geri-chair		E																															
Routine Resident Check Q 2 hrs.		N																															
		D																															
		E																															
Offered Fluids Q 2 hrs.		N																															
		D																															
		E																															
Linen Change T = Total P = Partial		N																															
		D																															
		E																															

NAME: _____   ROOM # _____

ADL FLOWSHEET

	HR	1	2	3	4	5	6	7	8	9	10	11	12	13	14	15	16	17	18	19	20	21	22	23	24	25	26	27	28	29	30	31
DIET:	B																															
75% (GOOD) 50% (FAIR) 25% (POOR)	L																															
S + SUBSTITUTE	D																															
( ) DINING ROOM ( ) FEEDS SELF	S																															
Bath ( ) Bed Bath (BB) ( ) Whirlpool (WP) ( ) Partial Bath (PB) ( ) Shower (S) ( ) Tub Bath (T B) ( ) Total Help (TH) ( ) Independent (I) ( ) Assistance (A)	D																															
	E																															
Oral Care ( ) Dentures	N																															
( ) Own Teeth ( ) Special Instructions	D																															
( ) Independent (I) ( ) Assistance (A) ( ) Total Help (TH)	E																															
Fingernail Care ( ) Independent (I) ( ) Assist (A) ( ) Total Help (TH) Toenail Care ( ) Independent (I) ( )Assist (A) ( ) Total Help (TH)	N																															
	N																															
Shave ( ) Independent (I) ( ) Assist (A) ( ) Total Help (TH) Shampoo ( ) Independent (I) ( ) Assist (A) ( ) Total Help (TH)	S																															
	S																															
Bowel Movement (BM)	N																															
	D																															
L = Large M = Medium S = Small	E																															
( ) Incontinent (I) ( ) Continent (C)	N																															
( ) Urine ( ) Incontinent (I) ( ) Continent (C)	D																															
( ) Feces ( ) Partial bath/Peri Care after each incontinent episode	E																															
Skin Care ( ) Turn and reposition Q2h	N																															
( ) Peri-Care ( ) Backrub	D																															
( ) Other: _____	E																															
Ambulation ( ) Ambulatory (I) ( ) Partial Bedfast	N																															
( ) Walker ( ) Geri-chair ( ) Cane ( ) Wheelchair	D																															
( ) Independent (I) ( ) Assist (A) ( ) Total Help (TH)	E																															
Protective Safety Device Q 1 hour, R/R Q 2 hours x 10 min. ( ) Vest ( ) Side Rails: _____	N																															
( ) Waist ( ) Geri-chair ( ) Lap Buddy ( ) Other: _____	D																															
_____	E																															
Routine Resident Check Q 2 hours ( )	N																															
Offered Fluids Q 2 hours ( )	D																															
	E																															
Linen Change	N																															
Total (T) Partial (P)	D																															
	E																															

RESIDENT NAME: _____   ROOM # _____

INTAKE-OUTPUT WORKSHEET

*Intake Equivalents

Medicine Cup—30 mL   Soup Bowl—8 oz./240 mL
Water Pitcher—800 mL/1000 mL   Ice Cream—3 oz./90 mL
Water Glass—8 oz./240 mL   Carton Milk—8 oz./240 mL
Styrofoam Cup (hot)—6 oz./180 mL
Juice Glass—4 oz./120 mL   *Chart in mL

TIME	INTAKE	OUTPUT	
	NOC	URINE	Emesis
			BM
			Drainage
	AM	URINE	Emesis
			BM
			Drainage
	PM	URINE	Emesis
			BM
			Drainage

INTAKE-OUTPUT WORKSHEET

*Intake Equivalents

Medicine Cup—30 mL   Soup Bowl—8 oz./240 mL
Water Pitcher—800 mL/1000 mL   Ice Cream—3 oz./90 mL
Water Glass—8 oz./240 mL   Carton Milk—8 oz./240 mL
Styrofoam Cup (hot)—6 oz./180 mL
Juice Glass—4 oz./120 mL   *Chart in mL

TIME	INTAKE	OUTPUT	
	NOC	URINE	Emesis
			BM
			Drainage
	AM	URINE	Emesis
			BM
			Drainage
	PM	URINE	Emesis
			BM
			Drainage

INTAKE-OUTPUT WORKSHEET

Intake Equivalents

Medicine Cup—30 mL	Soup Bowl 8 oz—240 mL	Water Pitcher—1000 mL
Water Glass 8 oz—240 mL	Styrofoam Cup 6 oz—180 mL	Juice Glass 4 oz—120 mL
Ice Cream 3 oz—90 mL	Carton Milk 8 oz—240 mL	Coffee Cup 6 oz—180 m L

Time	Intake	Output	
	NOC	URINE	EMESIS
			BM
			DRAINAGE

Time	Intake	Output	
	AM	URINE	EMESIS
			BM
			DRAINAGE

Time	Intake	Output	
	PM	URINE	EMESIS
			BM
			DRAINAGE

Measurements are guidelines only. Verify container size used in your facility.

RESIDENT: _____

ROOM:

_____

DATE: _____

INTAKE-OUTPUT WORKSHEET

Intake Equivalents

Medicine Cup—30 mL	Soup Bowl 8 oz—240 mL	Water Pitcher—1000 mL
Water Glass 8 oz—240 mL	Styrofoam Cup 6 oz—180 mL	Juice Glass 4 oz—120 mL
Ice Cream 3 oz—90 mL	Carton Milk 8 oz—240 mL	Coffee Cup 6 oz—180 m L

Time	Intake	Output	
	NOC	URINE	EMESIS
			BM
			DRAINAGE

Time	Intake	Output	
	AM	URINE	EMESIS
			BM
			DRAINAGE

Time	Intake	Output	
	PM	URINE	EMESIS
			BM
			DRAINAGE

Measurements are guidelines only. Verify container size used in your facility.

RESIDENT: _____

ROOM:

_____

DATE: _____

RESIDENT RESTRAINT RECORD

PHYSICIAN _____ RESIDENT _____

MONTH _____ YEAR _____ ROOM NO. _____

NA = NOT APPLICABLE	1	2	3	4	5	6	7	8	9	10	11	12	13	14	15	16	17	18	19	20	21	22	23	24	25	26	27	28	29	30	31
DAY																															
EVENING																															
NIGHT																															

DAY
TYPE OF RESTRAINT & REASON

EVENING
TYPE OF RESTRAINT & REASON

NIGHT
TYPE OF RESTRAINT & REASON

An initialed box on restraint record, for that shift indicates that the resident had position changed and personal needs met at least every two hours for ten minutes. For example: safety, range of motion, circulation, comfort, walked, incontinence, toileting needs, and other needs met. Restraints must be visually checked every 30 minutes for proper application and resident safety.

INITIALS	SIGNATURE	INITIALS	SIGNATURE	INITIALS	SIGNATURE	INITIALS	SIGNATURE

RESIDENT RESTRAINT RECORD

RESIDENT: _____

Month: _____ Year: _____

PHYSICIAN: _____ ROOM NO. _____

NA = NOT APPLICABLE	1	2	3	4	5	6	7	8	9	10	11	12	13	14	15	16	17	18	19	20	21	22	23	24	25	26	27	28	29	30	31
DAY																															
EVENING																															
NOC																															

DAY
TYPE OF RESTRAINT AND REASON

EVENING (PM)
TYPE OF RESTRAINT AND REASON

NIGHT (NOC)
TYPE OF RESTRAINT AND REASON

An initialed box on the restraint record for that shift indicates that the resident had position changed and personal needs met at least every two hours for ten minutes. For example: safety, range of motion, circulation, walked, toileted, incontinence care, and other needs met. Restraints must be visually checked every 30 minutes for proper application and resident safety.

INITIALS	SIGNATURE	INITIALS	SIGNATURE	INITIALS	SIGNATURE	INITIALS	SIGNATURE

DOCUMENTATION OF MEAL INTAKE

Date: _____

GUIDELINES FOR INTAKE:

Breakfast	All	3/4	1/2	1/4
Eggs	35%	25%	17%	9%
Milk	20%	15%	10%	5%
Juice	15%	12%	8%	4%
Toast/Biscuit	15%	12%	8%	4%
Cereal	15%	12%	8%	4%

Lunch & Supper	All	3/4	1/2	1/4
Meat or Sub.	50%	37%	25%	12%
Vegetable	15%	12%	8%	4%
Starch	5%	4%	3%	2%
Bread	5%	4%	3%	2%
Fruit	15%	12%	8%	4%
Fluids	10%	8%	5%	3%

BREAKFAST

NAME	eggs	milk	juice	toast	cereal	Total

LUNCH

meat	veg	starch	bread	dessert	fluids	Total

SUPPER

meat	veg	starch	bread	dessert	fluids	Total

DOCUMENTATION OF MEAL INTAKE   DATE: _____

GUIDELINES FOR INTAKE:

BREAKFAST	ALL	%	%	%
Eggs	35%	25%	17%	9%
Milk	20%	15%	10%	5%
Juice	15%	12%	8%	4%
Toast/Biscuit	15%	12%	8%	4%
Cereal	15%	12%	8%	4%

LUNCH AND DINNER	ALL	%	%	%
Meat or Substitute	50%	37%	25%	12%
Vegetable	15%	12%	8%	4%
Starch	5%	4%	3%	2%
Bread	5%	4%	3%	2%
Fruit	15%	12%	8%	4%
Fluids	10%	8%	5%	3%

BREAKFAST

NAME	meat	veg	starch	bread	dessert	fluids	total

LUNCH

	meat	veg	starch	bread	dessert	fluids	total

DINNER

	meat	veg	starch	bread	dessert	fluids	total

INITIAL INCONTINENCE EVALUATION (VOIDING PATTERN ASSESSMENT)

○ ○ ∅ ... incontinent SMALL amount ● Dry when checked

○ ∅ ○ ... incontinent MODERATE amount (/) Stool present

∅ ○ ○ ... incontinent LARGE amount (/) Resident asked to use toilet

Day _____ Date _____/_____/_____

NURSING ASSISTANT	TIME	INCONTINENT	DRY	STOOL	RESIDENT REQUESTED	TOILETED
	12 Midnite	○ ○ ○	●	( )	( )	mL
	1 AM	○ ○ ○	●	( )	( )	mL
	2 AM	○ ○ ○	●	( )	( )	mL
	3 AM	○ ○ ○	●	( )	( )	mL
	4 AM	○ ○ ○	●	( )	( )	mL
	5 AM	○ ○ ○	●	( )	( )	mL
	6 AM	○ ○ ○	●	( )	( )	mL
	7 AM	○ ○ ○	●	( )	( )	mL
	8 AM	○ ○ ○	●	( )	( )	mL
	9 AM	○ ○ ○	●	( )	( )	mL
	10 AM	○ ○ ○	●	( )	( )	mL
	11 AM	○ ○ ○	●	( )	( )	mL
	12 PM	○ ○ ○	●	( )	( )	mL
	1 PM	○ ○ ○	●	( )	( )	mL
	2 PM	○ ○ ○	●	( )	( )	mL
	3 PM	○ ○ ○	●	( )	( )	mL
	4 PM	○ ○ ○	●	( )	( )	mL
	5 PM	○ ○ ○	●	( )	( )	mL
	6 PM	○ ○ ○	●	( )	( )	mL
	7 PM	○ ○ ○	●	( )	( )	mL
	8 PM	○ ○ ○	●	( )	( )	mL
	9 PM	○ ○ ○	●	( )	( )	mL
	10 PM	○ ○ ○	●	( )	( )	mL
	11 PM	○ ○ ○	●	( )	( )	mL
TOTALS						mL

ESIDENT NAME: _____ ROOM NO. _____

INITIAL INCONTINENCE EVALUATION (VOIDING PATTERN ASSESSMENT)

○ ○ ⊘ — Incontinent **SMALL AMOUNT**

○ ⊘ ○ — Incontinent **MODERATE AMOUNT**

⊘ ○ ○ — Incontinent **LARGE AMOUNT**

●   **Dry when checked**

(/)   **Stool present**

(X)   **Resident asked to use toilet**

Day _____ Date _____/_____/_____

NURSING ASSISTANT	TIME	INCONTINENT	DRY	STOOL	RESIDENT REQUESTED	TOILETED
	12 MIDNIGHT	○ ○ ○	●	( )	( )	mL
	1 AM	○ ○ ○	●	( )	( )	mL
	2 AM	○ ○ ○	●	( )	( )	mL
	3 AM	○ ○ ○	●	( )	( )	mL
	4 AM	○ ○ ○	●	( )	( )	mL
	5 AM	○ ○ ○	●	( )	( )	mL
	6 AM	○ ○ ○	●	( )	( )	mL
	7 AM	○ ○ ○	●	( )	( )	mL
	8 AM	○ ○ ○	●	( )	( )	mL
	9 AM	○ ○ ○	●	( )	( )	mL
	10 AM	○ ○ ○	●	( )	( )	mL
	11 AM	○ ○ ○	●	( )	( )	mL
	12 PM	○ ○ ○	●	( )	( )	mL
	1 PM	○ ○ ○	●	( )	( )	mL
	2 PM	○ ○ ○	●	( )	( )	mL
	3 PM	○ ○ ○	●	( )	( )	mL
	4 PM	○ ○ ○	●	( )	( )	mL
	5 PM	○ ○ ○	●	( )	( )	mL
	6 PM	○ ○ ○	●	( )	( )	mL
	7 PM	○ ○ ○	●	( )	( )	mL
	8 PM	○ ○ ○	●	( )	( )	mL
	9 PM	○ ○ ○	●	( )	( )	mL
	10 PM	○ ○ ○	●	( )	( )	mL
	11 PM	○ ○ ○	●	( )	( )	mL
TOTALS						mL

RESIDENT NAME: _____ ROOM NO. _____

ASSESSMENT FOR BOWEL AND BLADDER TRAINING

RESIDENT _____ ROOM NO _____

	DAY 1	DAY 2	DAY 3	DAY 4	DAY 5	DAY 6	DAY 7
DATE							
7 AM							
8 AM							
9 AM							
10 AM							
11 AM							
12 PM							
1 PM							
2 PM							
3 PM							
4 PM							
5 PM							
6 PM							
7 PM							
8 PM							
9 PM							
10 PM							
11 PM							
12 AM							
1 AM							
2 AM							
3 AM							
4 AM							
5 AM							
6 AM							
CODE:	D = DRY		TBM = TOILET BM				
	IBM = INCONTINENT BM		TU = TOILET URINE				
	IU = INCONTINENT URINE						

ASSESSMENT FOR BOWEL AND BLADDER TRAINING

Resident _____ Room No _____

	DAY 1	DAY 2	DAY 3	DAY 4	DAY 5	DAY 6	DAY 7
DATE							
6 AM							
7 AM							
8 AM							
9 AM							
10 AM							
11 AM							
12 PM							
1 PM							
2 PM							
3 PM							
4 PM							
5 PM							
6 PM							
7 PM							
8 PM							
9 PM							
10 PM							
11 PM							
12 AM							
1 AM							
2 AM							
3 AM							
4 AM							
5 AM							

CODE:
D = DRY
TU = TOILET URINE   TBM = TOILET BM
IU = INCONTINENT URINE IBM = INCONTINENT BM

WEIGHT RECORD

DATE	WEIGHT WT	HEIGHT HT	COMMENTS/SIGNATURE	DATE	WEIGHT WT	COMMENTS/SIGNATURE
			ON ADMISSION			

LAST NAME, FIRST NAME, & INITIAL	ATTENDING PHYSICIAN	ROOM NO.	RESIDENT NO.

WEIGHT RECORD

DATE	WT	HT	COMMENTS/ SIGNATURE	DATE	WT	COMMENTS/ SIGNATURE
			ON ADMISSION			

LAST NAME, FIRST NAME, INITIAL	PHYSICIAN	ROOM NO.	RESIDENT NO.

VITAL SIGN RECORD

DATE	TEMPERATURE T	PULSE P	RESPIRATION R	BLOOD PRESSURE BP	SHIFT	COMMENTS	DATE	TEMPERATURE T	PULSE P	RESPIRATION R	BLOOD PRESSURE BP	SHIFT	COMMENTS

IF PULSE IS APICAL - PRECEDE RECORDING WITH LETTER "A"

LAST NAME, FIRST NAME & INITIAL	ATTENDING PHYSICIAN	ROOM NO.	RESIDENT NO.

VITAL SIGN RECORD

DATE	T	P	R	B/P	SHIFT	COMMENTS	DATE	T	P	R	B/P	SHIFT	COMMENTS

LAST NAME, FIRST NAME, INITIAL	PHYSICIAN	ROOM NO.	RESIDENT NO.

IMPRINT AREA

GRAPHIC RECORD

		12	4	8	12	4	8	12	4	8	12	4	8	12	4	8	12	4	8	12	4	8	12	4	8	12	4	8	12	4	8	12	4	8	12	4	8
DATE																																					
HOSPITAL DAY																																					
POST OP DAY																																					
TIME		12	4	8	12	4	8	12	4	8	12	4	8	12	4	8	12	4	8	12	4	8	12	4	8	12	4	8	12	4	8	12	4	8	12	4	8

TEMPERATURE
105° 104° 103° 102° 101° 100° 99° 98° 97°

PULSE
170 160 150 140 130 120 110 100 90 80 70 60

RESPIRATION
50 40 30 20 10

BLOOD PRESSURE	A M	12	4	8	12	4	8	12	4	8	12	4	8	12	4	8	12	4	8
	P M	12	4	8	12	4	8	12	4	8	12	4	8	12	4	8	12	4	8

WEIGHT	STOOL							

QTY.	ARTICLES	3	ITEMS OF SPECIFIC VALUE (RINGS, WATCHES, RADIOS, ETC.)		3

RESIDENT NAME

INVENTORY OF PERSONAL EFFECTS

ROOM NO.

DATE OF INVENTORY

QTY.	ARTICLES	3	DESCRIPTION	VALUE	3
	DRESSES			$	
	LADIES SUITS				
	COATS				
	FURS				
	LADIES SHOES				
	LADIES HATS				
	BLOUSES				
	LADIES SWEATERS				
	GLOVES				
	HOSE				
	LADIES HANDKERCHIEFS				
	SLIPS				
	FOUNDATION GARMENTS		ACQUIRED AFTER ORIGINAL ENTRY		3
	BRASSIERES		DATE · ITEM · HOW RECEIVED		
	NIGHTGOWNS				
	HOUSECOATS - ROBES				
	HOUSE SLIPPERS				
	POCKET BOOKS				
	OVERNIGHT CASE				
	MEN'S SUITS				
	TOPCOATS				
	SLACKS				
	SPORTS JACKETS				
	MEN'S HATS				
	MEN'S SHOES				
	MEN'S GLOVES				
	SOCKS				
	SHORTS				
	UNDERSHIRTS				
	TIES				
	BELTS - SUSPENDERS		NOTES ON ARTICLES		
	MEN'S HANDKERCHIEFS		(LISTING OF ITEMS DAMAGED, LOST, ETC.)		
	PAJAMAS				
	ROBES				
	SLIPPERS				
	SHAVING KIT				
	TRAVELING BAGS				
	HEARING AID				
	DENTURES				
	GLASSES				
	OTHER:				

REMARKS:

CERTIFICATION OF RECEIPT

ON ADMISSION	ON DISCHARGE
SIGNED	SIGNED
_____	_____
(RESIDENT OR RESPONSIBLE PARTY) DATE	(RESIDENT OR RESPONSIBLE PARTY) DATE
SIGNED	SIGNED
_____	_____
TITLE DATE	TITLE DATE

Source: Courtesy of Briggs Corporation, Des Moines IA (800) 247-2343

SEVEN-DAY RESIDENT SELF-ABILITY EVALUATION

Instructions: For each shift, enter the appropriate number in the space provided.
Document the resident's ability to perform those areas listed.

1 = self able totally indep
2 = self able with setup
3 = self able with one
4 = self able limited
5 = self able not possible

	Date			Date			Date			Date			Date			Date			Date		
	D	E	N	D	E	N	D	E	N	D	E	N	D	E	N	D	E	N	D	E	N
Bathing Shower [ ] Tub [ ]																					
Body Alignment																					
Dressing [includes appliances]																					
Toilet Use [transfer, use of appliances]																					
Grooming [nails, hair, face]																					
Ambulation [include use of wheelchair, walker, etc.]																					
Transfer Ability																					
Eating Tube feeding [ ] enter T																					
CNA Initial																					

CNA Signatures

_____   _____   _____

_____   _____   _____

_____   _____   _____

_____   _____   _____

SUMMARY OF RESIDENT'S ABILITY TO SELF-PERFORM ADL ACTIVITIES—7 DAYS:

_____   _____
              Nurse   **Date**

Resident		**Rm/Bd**	**Physician**

SEVEN-DAY RESIDENT SELF-ABILITY EVALUATION

INSTRUCTIONS: For each shift, enter the appropriate number in the spaces provided.
Document the resident's ability to perform those areas listed.

1 = self able totally Indep 2 = self able with setup 3 = self able with one 4 = self able limited 5 = self able not possible		Date			Date			Date			Date			Date			Date			Date		
		D	E	N	D	E	N	D	E	N	D	E	N	D	E	N	D	E	N	D	E	N
Bathing Shower ( ) Tub ( )																							
Body Alignment																							
Dressing (Includes appliances)																							
Toilet Use (Includes transfer, use of appliances)																							
Grooming (Nails, hair, face)																							
Ambulation (Includes use of wheelchair, walker, etc.)																							
Transfer Ability																							
Eating Tube feeding enter (T)																							
CNA Initials																							

CNA Signatures

------------------------------   ------------------------------   ------------------------------

------------------------------   ------------------------------   ------------------------------

------------------------------   ------------------------------   ------------------------------

------------------------------   ------------------------------   ------------------------------

SUMMARY OF RESIDENT'S ABILITY TO SELF-PERFORM ADL ACTIVITIES—7 DAYS:

---------------------------------------   ---------------------------------------
Nurse   **Date**

Resident	Room/Bed	Physician

RM _____ NAME _____
Ate _____ % Brk _____ BM
Ate _____ % Lch _____ SBM
Ate _____ % Sup _____ MBM
Shower _____ Bed-bath _____ LBM
Intake _____ mL _____ Change
Output _____ mL Oral _____ R _____ Ax
Temp _____ Oral _____ R _____ Ax
Pulse _____ Resp _____
Wt. _____ BP _____
Sp Inst:

(This block is repeated across eleven cells of the worksheet grid.)

NURSING ASSISTANT RESIDENT CARE WORKSHEET

Signature Nurse: _____
Nursing Assistant: _____

DATE: _____ SHIFT _____ HALL # _____
(Keep for 30 days.)
(Signature certifies that all assignments noted have been completed.)

RM _____ NAME __________
Ate _____% Brk
Ate _____% Lch
Ate _____% Sup
Shower Bedbath LBM
Intake ______ mL Linen
Change ______
Output ______ mL
Temp _____ Oral R Ax
Pulse _____ Resp _____
BP _______ Wt _____
Sp Inst:
____
____
____
____

RM _____ NAME __________
Ate _____% Brk
Ate _____% Lch
Ate _____% Sup
Shower Bedbath LBM
Intake ______ mL Linen
Change ______
Output ______ mL
Temp _____ Oral R Ax
Pulse _____ Resp _____
BP _______ Wt _____
Sp Inst:
____
____
____
____

RM _____ NAME __________
Ate _____% Brk
Ate _____% Lch
Ate _____% Sup
Shower Bedbath LBM
Intake ______ mL Linen
Change ______
Output ______ mL
Temp _____ Oral R Ax
Pulse _____ Resp _____
BP _______ Wt _____
Sp Inst:
____
____
____
____

RM _____ NAME __________
Ate _____% Brk
Ate _____% Lch
Ate _____% Sup
Shower Bedbath LBM
Intake ______ mL Linen
Change ______
Output ______ mL
Temp _____ Oral R Ax
Pulse _____ Resp _____
BP _______ Wt _____
Sp Inst:
____
____
____
____

RM _____ NAME __________
Ate _____% Brk
Ate _____% Lch
Ate _____% Sup
Shower Bedbath LBM
Intake ______ mL Linen
Change ______
Output ______ mL
Temp _____ Oral R Ax
Pulse _____ Resp _____
BP _______ Wt _____
Sp Inst:
____
____
____
____

RM _____ NAME __________
Ate _____% Brk
Ate _____% Lch
Ate _____% Sup
Shower Bedbath LBM
Intake ______ mL Linen
Change ______
Output ______ mL
Temp _____ Oral R Ax
Pulse _____ Resp _____
BP _______ Wt _____
Sp Inst:
____
____
____
____

RM _____ NAME __________
Ate _____% Brk
Ate _____% Lch
Ate _____% Sup
Shower Bedbath LBM
Intake ______ mL Linen
Change ______
Output ______ mL
Temp _____ Oral R Ax
Pulse _____ Resp _____
BP _______ Wt _____
Sp Inst:
____
____
____
____

RM _____ NAME __________
Ate _____% Brk
Ate _____% Lch
Ate _____% Sup
Shower Bedbath LBM
Intake ______ mL Linen
Change ______
Output ______ mL
Temp _____ Oral R Ax
Pulse _____ Resp _____
BP _______ Wt _____
Sp Inst:
____
____
____
____

RM _____ NAME __________
Ate _____% Brk
Ate _____% Lch
Ate _____% Sup
Shower Bedbath LBM
Intake ______ mL Linen
Change ______
Output ______ mL
Temp _____ Oral R Ax
Pulse _____ Resp _____
BP _______ Wt _____
Sp Inst:
____
____
____
____

RM _____ NAME __________
Ate _____% Brk
Ate _____% Lch
Ate _____% Sup
Shower Bedbath LBM
Intake ______ mL Linen
Change ______
Output ______ mL
Temp _____ Oral R Ax
Pulse _____ Resp _____
BP _______ Wt _____
Sp Inst:
____
____
____
____

RM _____ NAME __________
Ate _____% Brk
Ate _____% Lch
Ate _____% Sup
Shower Bedbath LBM
Intake ______ mL Linen
Change ______
Output ______ mL
Temp _____ Oral R Ax
Pulse _____ Resp _____
BP _______ Wt _____
Sp Inst:
____
____
____
____

RM _____ NAME __________
Ate _____% Brk
Ate _____% Lch
Ate _____% Sup
Shower Bedbath LBM
Intake ______ mL Linen
Change ______
Output ______ mL
Temp _____ Oral R Ax
Pulse _____ Resp _____
BP _______ Wt _____
Sp Inst:
____
____
____
____

RM _____ NAME __________
Ate _____% Brk
Ate _____% Lch
Ate _____% Sup
Shower Bedbath LBM
Intake ______ mL Linen
Change ______
Output ______ mL
Temp _____ Oral R Ax
Pulse _____ Resp _____
BP _______ Wt _____
Sp Inst:
____
____
____
____

Resident Care Worksheet

Signature Nurse:

____

Nursing Assistants:

____

____

____

____

DATE: ____________ **SHIFT** _________ **HALL #** _________

(Keep for 30 days.)

(Signature certifies that all assignments noted have been completed.)

NURSING ASSISTANT ASSIGNMENT SHEET

A# _____

TURN IN TO NURSE BY _____   AM/PM _____

NURSING ASSISTANT NAME _____

SPECIAL ASSIGNMENT _____

NURSE _____   BREAK _____   MEAL _____   SHIFT _____

DATE _____   BREAK _____   MEAL _____   SHIFT _____

RM	Name	Activity Status	Snack/ Supplement A/R	Oral Care	Bath	Shampoo	Nail Care	Shave	Incontinent Foley Output- Continent	B.M.	Restraint Type ck. q 30 min. R&R q 2 hrs. x 10 min.	Special Care and/or Remarks

☐ Linen Room   ☐ Clean Shower Room   ☐ Assist Hall Trays
☐ Pass Fresh Drinking Water/Ice   ☐ Assist Dining Room   ☐ Monitor Halls
☐ Clean Utility Closet   ☐ Relieve NA # _____   ☐ Feed Hall Trays

Signature _____ Nursing Assistant

NURSING ASSISTANT ASSIGNMENT SHEET

TURN IN TO CHARGE NURSE BY _____ AM/PM

SPECIAL ASSIGNMENT _____

| | BREAK _____ | MEAL _____ | SHIFT _____ |
| | BREAK _____ | MEAL _____ | SHIFT _____ |

NURSING ASSISTANT NAME _____

CHARGE NURSE _____

DATE _____

RM	NAME	Activity Status	Snack/ Supplement	Oral Care	Bath	Shampoo	Nail Care	Shave	Incontinent Foley/Output Continent	BM	Restraint Type	Special Care and/or Remarks

☐ Linen Room   ☐ Clean Shower Room   ☐ Assist Hall Trays
☐ Pass Drinking Water/Ice   ☐ Assist Dining Room   ☐ Monitor Halls
☐ Clean Utility Closet   ☐ Relieve NA # _____   ☐ Feed Hall Trays

Signature _____ Nursing Assistant

NURSING ASSISTANT COMMUNICATION LOG

NA Name: _____   Resident Name: _____   Date: _____

Time	T	P	R	B/P	Mark Skin Problems on Diagram
Height	**Weight**				

Elimination					
Urination	Continent	Incontinent	How Many?	Abnormalities	
BM-Large	BM-Medium	BM-Small	No BM	Abnormalities	

Indicate Ulcer Sites

Anterior   Posterior

General Information	
Bath	
Nails done	
Oral care	
Skin condition-Be specific! (hydrated, abnormalities, etc.)	
Assistance with ambulation	
Protective safety device (if any) applied and released	

(Attach a color photo of the pressure ulcer(s) [optonal])

Fluid Consumption				
Good	Fair	Poor	Intake, if ordered	Output, if ordered

Meal Consumption (Circle One)					
Breakfast	Good	Fair	Poor	Substitute?	Refused/Comment
Lunch	Good	Fair	Poor	Substitute?	Refused/Comment
AM Snack	Good	Fair	Poor	Refused	Comment
PM Snack	Good	Fair	Poor	Refused	Comment

Attitude/Mental Condition (Circle One)				Comments, Concerns, Issues to Report to Nurse
Sad	Happy	Sleepy	Other (Specify)	
Comment:				
Activities, if any				

Nurse/CNA Communication Log

Nursing Assistant: **Date:**

6–2							2–10						
Vital Signs:							Vital Signs:						
Time	T	P	R	B/P	02	RSI	Time	T	P	R	B/P	02	RSI

BMs		BMs	

General Info	General Info

OOB:	**OOB:**
PT Programs:	**PT Programs:**
ROM	**ROM**
Ambulate	**Ambulate**
AFOs On	**AFOs On**
Body Jacket On	**Body Jacket On**
OT Programs:	**OT Programs:**
Oral Stim	**Oral Stim**
Hand Splints On	**Hand Splints On**
Feeding Issues:	**Feeding Issues:**

Meal Consumption:
Good   Fair   Poor
Good   Fair   Poor

Fluid Consumption:
Good   Fair   Poor
Good   Fair   Poor

Menses:
Heavy   Moderate   Light   Scant

HS:

Meal Consumption:
Good   Fair   Poor
Good   Fair   Poor

Fluid Consumption:
Good   Fair   Poor
Good   Fair   Poor

Menses:
Heavy   Moderate   Light   Scant

HS:

Other Info (Phone calls, behaviors)	Other Info (Phone calls, behaviors)

Nursing Assistant Performance Record

Nursing Assistant Name (Last, First)   Social Security Number

(Program Name, Location)

Dates of Class ____/____/____ to ____/____/____   S = Satisfactory Performance
                mm   dd   yyyy   mm   dd   yyyy

                                                          U = Unsatisfactory Performance

                                                          ★ = See comments

☆ **Program Code Number** ☆   Ints. = Initials

Place a full signature here to correspond with each set of initials on the form.

Initials	Corresponding Signature of Instructor	Title

No.	PROCEDURAL GUIDELINES	CLASSROOM			SKILLS LAB			CLINICAL		
		S/U	Date	Ints.	S/U	Date	Ints.	S/U	Date	Ints.

Feel free to duplicate the performance record. Fill in the skills the student has completed. Retain the original in the master class file.

Nursing Assistant Performance Record *(continued)*

No.	PROCEDURAL GUIDELINES	CLASSROOM			SKILLS LAB			CLINICAL		
		S/U	Date	Ints.	S/U	Date	Ints.	S/U	Date	Ints.

Feel free to duplicate the performance record. Fill in the skills the student has completed. Retain the original in the master class file.

Nursing Assistant Performance Record *(continued)*

No.	PROCEDURAL GUIDELINES	CLASSROOM			SKILLS LAB			CLINICAL		
		S/U	Date	Ints.	S/U	Date	Ints.	S/U	Date	Ints.

Feel free to duplicate the performance record. Fill in the skills the student has completed. Retain the original in the master class file.

Nursing Assistant Performance Review Checklist

_____   _____
Nursing Assistant Name (Last, First)   **Student Identification Number**

_____
Procedure Name and Number

S   = Satisfactory Performance
U   = Unsatisfactory Performance
★   = See comments
Ints. = Initials

Place a full signature here to correspond with each set of initials on the form.

Initials	Corresponding Signature of Instructor	Title

No.	PROCEDURAL GUIDELINES	CLASSROOM			SKILLS LAB			CLINICAL		
		S/U	Date	Ints.	S/U	Date	Ints.	S/U	Date	Ints.

Feel free to duplicate the performance record. Fill in the skills the student has completed. Retain the original in the master class file.

Nursing Assistant Performance Review Checklist *(continued)*

No.	PROCEDURAL GUIDELINES	CLASSROOM			SKILLS LAB			CLINICAL		
		S/U	Date	Ints.	S/U	Date	Ints.	S/U	Date	Ints.

Comments:

_____

_____

_____

_____

_____

_____

_____

_____

_____

_____

_____

_____

_____

_____

Feel free to duplicate the performance record. Fill in the skills the student has completed. Retain the original in the master class file.

Page 2 of 2

PART V

Flash Cards

1x, 2x, etc.	one time, one person, two times, etc.
$\overline{a}$	before
@	at
ad lib	as desired
ADLs	activities of daily living
aka	above-the-knee amputation; also known as
am	morning
AMA	against medical advice
amb	ambulate
amt	amount
ant	anterior
AROM	active range of motion
ASAP	as soon as possible
assist	assistance
as tol	as tolerated
az, (A)	axillary (under the arm)
B, (B), Ⓑ	bilateral, both

B&B	bowel and bladder
BB	bed bath
bid	twice a day
bil, bilat	bilateral
BKA	below-the-knee amputation
BLE	both lower extremites
BM	bowel movement
BP *or* B/P	blood pressure
BPM	beats per minute
BR, B/R	bedrest, bathroom
BRP	bathroom privileges
BSC	bedside commode
BUE	both upper extremites
$\overline{c}$	with
cc	cubic centimeter
cath	catheter
CBB	complete bed bath

ck or ✔	check
ck or ✔ freq	check frequently
cl liq	clear liquid
cm	centimeter
CNA	certified nursing assistant
c/o	complains of
COLD, COPD	chronic obstructive lung (pulmonary) disease
CP	care plan, chest pain (in context)
CPR	cardiopulmonary resuscitation
C & S	culture and sensitivity
CVA	cerebrovascular accident, stroke
CXR	chest x-ray
D/C, DC	discontinue, discharge
diab	diabetes, diabetic
DNR	do not resuscitate
ESRD	end-stage renal disease
et	and

F	Fahrenheit, fair (in context)
FF	force fluids
freq	frequently
Fx	fracture
g/c, GC	geriatric chair
G/T, GT	gastrostomy tube
H_2O	water
H_2O_2	hydrogen peroxide
HOB	head of bed
HOH	hard of hearing
hr	hour
hs	bedtime (hour of sleep)
ht	height
Ⓘ, ind.	independent, independently
I & O	intake and output
isol	isolation
IV	intravenous

L	liter
LA	left arm
lab	laboratory
lat	lateral
lb	pound
LE	lower extremity
LL	left leg
LLE	left lower extremity
lg	large
liq	liquid
L/min *or* LPM	liters per minute
LOC	loss of consciousness, level of consciousness, level of care
L, lt	left
max	maximum
mech soft	mechanical soft
min	minimum, minimal, minute

mL *or* ml	milliliter
mm	millimeter
mmHg	millimeters of mercury
mod	moderate
MRSA	methicillin-resistant Staphylococcus aureus
NAR	no adverse reaction
NAS	no added salt
N/C	no complaints
neg *or* −	negative
NG	nasogastric
NIDDM	noninsulin-dependent diabetes mellitus
NKA	no known allergies
noc	night
NPA	nothing by mouth
N/S, NSS	normal saline
N & V	nausea and vomiting

NWB	non-weight bearing
obs	observations
occ	occasional
O_2	oxygen
OOB	out of bed
ORIF	open reduction, internal fixation
os, (O)	mouth
oz	ounce
$\bar{p}$	after
PB, PBB	partial bath, partial bed bath
$\overline{pc}$	after meals
per	by, through
pm	afternoon or evening
po	by mouth
pos *or* +	positive
prn	as needed
PROM	passive range of motion

pt *or* Pt	patient
PWB	partial weight bearing
q̄	each, every
q2h, q3h, q4h, etc.	every two hours, every three hours, every four hours, etc.
qid	four times a day
qs	sufficient quantity
qt	quart
quad	quadrant, quadriplegic
R	rectal, respiration, right
RA	rheumatoid arthritis, right arm
reg	regular
reps	repetitions
res *or* Res	resident
resp, R	respirations
RL	right leg
RLE	right lower extremity

RLQ	right lower quadrant
rm	room
rt	related to
RUE	right upper extremity
RUQ	right upper quadrant
Rx	prescription, therapy, treatment
$\bar{s}$	without
SBA	standby assistance
sm	small
SOB	shortness of breath
spec	specimen
S/T	skin tear
stat	immediately
T, temp	temperature
TB	tuberculosis
TF	tube feeding
TID	three times a day

TPR	temperature, pulse, respiration
trach	tracheostomy
UA *or* U/A	urinalysis
UE	upper extremity
URI	upper respiratory infection
UTI	urinary tract infection
vag	vaginal
vc, VC	verbal cues
VRE	vancomycin-resistant Enterococcus
VS	vital signs
WA *or* W/A	while awake
WB	weight bearing
WBAT	weight bearing as tolerated
w/c	wheelchair
WFL	within functional limits
WNL	within normal limits
wt	weight

x _or_ X	times
↑	up, increase
↓	down, decrease
=	equals, equal to
> _or_ ≥	greater than
< _or_ ≤	less than
± _or_ +/−	plus or minus
Δ	change to, change in
°	degrees
Ø	zero, none, nothing
1x	one time, one person
2°	secondary to
*	important